To all those interested in improving their health I
can't recommend Dr Myhill's *PK Cookbook* highly
a number of years and had failed to see any imp
conventional medical approaches. I was therefore
books all of which I found to be extremely informat
ous scientific studies and incredibly readable (and
hours of commencing the PK diet, symptoms that I'd had for years (headaches/
migraines and gastrointestinal pain) resolved completely. Friends and family that
I subsequently encouraged to also convert to a PK diet have enjoyed improve-
ments in a range of health conditions including obesity, obstructive sleep apnoea,
hypertension, recalcitrant skin problems, anxiety symptoms and IBS to name but
a few. Starting the PK diet may seem daunting at first as it's significantly different
from the standard western diet but Dr Myhill's *PK Cookbook* is incredibly easy to
follow such that the nutritional changes soon become second-nature – and the
recipes and meal ideas are delicious too. So my advice to anyone who's contem-
plating the PK diet is simple – benefit from Dr Myhill's years of experience and
wealth of knowledge, take control of your own health and GO FOR IT!

Dr Christopher Afford MA MB BChir (Cantab) MRCS (Eng)

Although I knew intellectually that the Paleo-Ketogenic diet was what I should
be doing, the prospect of attempting it was really daunting. I wouldn't even have
attempted it without Dr Myhill's book, which anticipated my concerns and guided
me through what I thought was going to be a difficult journey. It described exactly
what to expect and how to know when one has arrived; I found it so much easier
than I expected. The meal suggestions and recipes are quick and easy, but more importantly are tasty, substantial and filling. The bread and dairy alternatives mean
that I can entertain friends at home without them realising that they are eating a
PK meal. Within just a few days of starting the PK diet, I was surprised to find that
my long term reflux symptoms had completely resolved. I had resigned myself to
lifelong reflux medication, which had already contributed to osteopenia (thinning
of my bones), but now I am delighted that I no longer need it. I am confident that
this is a way of eating that I shall stick to for the rest of my life.

Dr Rowena Nicholson MB BS MRCGP
General Practitioner

We've known Sarah for more than 20 years, both as a doctor to our daughter and
now as a trusted friend. Her work has done much to help our daughter through
many difficult times. It is well researched, simple to understand, and what's more,
effective. We have read and used her *Prevent and Cure Diabetes* book and have no
hesitation in recommending this new work. We thank her for it and you will too.
    Sarah is a force of nature… It must be down to what she eats!

Jules, Diana and Ellie Nancarrow
Patients

This is a well written, comprehensive guide to the principles of the PK diet, full of tips and ideas with delicious and satisfying health-improvement plans that can be easily implemented. I appreciated being able to start the PK diet with a 'no-cook no-preparation' approach followed by introducing PK bread and salts. This diet will definitely be the foundation of my long-term health plan.

Olga Cary BA Dip CG
Patient

the PK
COOKBOOK

Go Paleo-ketogenic and get the best of both worlds

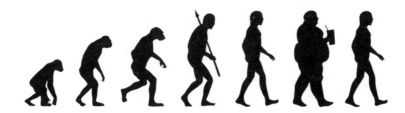

Dr Sarah Myhill MB BS and Craig Robinson MA (Oxon)

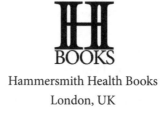

BOOKS

Hammersmith Health Books
London, UK

First published in 2017 by Hammersmith Health Books
– an imprint of Hammersmith Books Limited
4/4A Bloomsbury Square, London WC1A 2RP, UK
www.hammersmithbooks.co.uk

Reprinted 2018, 2019

The information contained in this book is for educational purposes only. It is the result of
the study and the experience of the authors. Whilst the information and advice offered
are believed to be true and accurate at the time of going to press, neither the authors
nor the publisher can accept any legal responsibility or liability for any errors or omis-
sions that may have been made or for any adverse effects which may occur as a result
of following the recommendations given herein. Always consult a qualified medical
practitioner if you have any concerns regarding your health.

British Library Cataloguing in Publication Data: A CIP record of this book is available
from the British Library.

Print ISBN 978-1-78161-128-9
Ebook ISBN 978-1-78161-129-6

Commissioning editor: Georgina Bentliff
Designed and typeset by: Julie Bennett, Bespoke Publishing Ltd
Cover design by: Sylvia Kwan
Index: Dr Laurence Errington
Production: Helen Whitehorn, Path Projects Ltd
Printed and bound by: TJ International Ltd
Cover illustration: Sanchez Cotan, Juan (1560-1627): Still Life with Game Fowl, 1600-1603
Chicago (IL) Art Institute of Chicago ©Photo SCALA, Florence, Italy, 2017

Contents

About the authors

Dr Sarah Myhill MB BS qualified in medicine (with Honours) from Middlesex Hospital Medical School in 1981 and has since focused tirelessly on identifying and treating the underlying causes of health problems, especially the 'diseases of civilisation' with which we are beset in the West. She has worked in the NHS and private practice and for 17 years was the Hon. Secretary of the British Society for Ecological Medicine, which focuses on the causes of disease and treating through diet, supplements and avoiding toxic stress. She helps to run and lectures at the Society's training courses and also lectures regularly on organophosphate poisoning, the problems of silicone, and chronic fatigue syndrome. Visit her website at www.drmyhill.co.uk

Craig Robinson MA took a first in Mathematics at Oxford University in 1985. He then joined Price Waterhouse and qualified as a Chartered Accountant in 1988, after which he worked as a lecturer in the private sector, and also in The City of London, primarily in Financial Sector Regulation roles. Craig first met Sarah in 2001, as a patient for the treatment of his CFS, and since then they have developed a professional working relationship, where he helps with the maintenance of www.drmyhill.co.uk, the moderating of Dr Myhill's Facebook groups and other ad hoc projects, as well as with the editing and writing of her books.

Stylistic note: Use of the first person singular in this book refers to me, Dr Sarah Myhill. One can assume that the medicine and biochemistry are mine, as edited by Craig Robinson, and that the classical and mathematical references are Craig's.

Dedication

SM: 'To my lovely patients, who have been willing guinea pigs and most forgiving when my suggestions have not worked. However, in doing so, they have pushed forward the frontiers of practical medicine.'

CR: 'To my Mum and Dad. From Mum I learned the power of imagination and wonderment, and to take your own path. From Dad I learned that if a job is worth doing, then it is worth doing well.'

Introduction
What is the PK diet?

The PK diet is a *combination* of the paleo diet (that which humans evolved into eating over a period of 2.5 million years) and the ketogenic diet.

In the Table on page xi we compare the pros and cons of nine different diets, including the PK diet, in order to demonstrate why this has the most significant health benefits.

'The combination is more than the sum of its pieces'

better known as:

'The whole is greater than the sum of its parts.'

Aristotle, 384 – 322 BC

The paleo or Stone Age diet

Of course, in Paleolithic, pre-agricultural times there was no single diet – local conditions would have dictated what could be foraged and hunted. The constant factor would have been that no foods were cultivated. However, at the present time we use 'paleo diet' to denote one that consists of natural, unprocessed foods and rejects grains and dairy. Proportions of macronutrients (carbohydrates, protein and fats) within this diet are not part of the definition.

The ketogenic diet

The body is remarkably adept at obtaining its fuels from a variety of foods. Carbohydrates are not essential foods – we can survive without them. The fuel which actually enters our mitochondria (the power houses of all our cells) is acetate. One can get to acetate from fat via ketones and from fermenting vegetable fibre in the gut via short-chain fatty acids as well as from carbohydrates and proteins via glucose. The ketogenic diet is one that results in the metabolic state whereby the majority of the body's energy is derived from ketone bodies in the blood – the state of 'ketosis'. This is in contrast to the state of glycolysis where blood glucose provides the majority of the energy supply. A person who is 'keto-adapted' is able to switch from burning sugar and carbs as a source of fuel to burning fat and fibre, which gives much longer lasting energy and stamina, of which more later. (Ketogenic diets have been shown to have remarkable benefits for a number of serious health problems, including epilepsy. The foods used in these medicinal diets tend to be highly processed.)

The combination

The addition of the ketogenic approach to the paleo diet has become necessary because modern paleo diets may be high in carbs and ignore the seasons. Whilst autumn paleo would have included fruits, honey, grains, nuts and pulses, these foods would have been absent for winter, spring and most of summer. During the winter, primitive man would have relied on meat, seafood and the accompanying fats as his staple foods – in other words, a ketogenic diet. To make use of this, he would have needed the ability to burn fats as the body's principal fuel.

'To everything there is a season…'

Ecclesiastes 3, King James V version, *The Bible*

The PK diet reflects the importance of burning fats and short-chain fatty acids as well as, or instead of, sugars, and the ability to swap between these options. What this means in practice is that the occasional seasonal excursion into autumn delights will do little harm to our health. Constant 'autumn mode' is fine in the short term, but damaging to health in the long term. Long-term 'autumn mode' results in metabolic syndrome – the loss of control of blood sugar that precedes the onset of type-2 diabetes. There is much more detail on this in our book *Prevent and Cure Diabetes – delicious diets not dangerous drugs* which gives the *why* of the ketogenic diet. This *PK Cookbook* delivers the *how*.

What follows in this book is what we should all be doing for *most* of the time – and as we age, we should spend more time in 'winter eating mode'. This is because as we grow older, our internal metabolism becomes less efficient. Like an old car, we need the best possible fuel and regular servicing. So, for example, our ability to digest and absorb foods well and our ability to produce hormones (such as the adrenal and thyroid hormones) declines, so we must box clever and help our bodies as much as possible, not only to live long but also to stay healthy into our mature years, and so 'live well'.

'*Dum vivimus vivamus*' – '*While we live, let us live!*'
The motto of Philip Doddridge's (26 June 1702 – 26 October 1751) coat of arms.
(Doddridge was an English nonconformist leader, educator and hymn writer.)

Table 1.1 summarises the pros and cons of nine commonly used but different types of diet – the 'standard Western', the paleo, the ketogenic, low-fat slimming diets, GAPS, vegetarian, vegan, allergy exclusion and PK.

Table 1: Comparison of diets

Diet	Pros	Cons	Notes: See our book *Prevent and Cure Diabetes* for details of all the below.
'Standard Western'	Westerners no longer suffer from starvation, but this diet has little else to commend it	High in refined carbohydrates such as sugar, fruit and fruit juice, potato, cereal, grains, and 'junk food'	Induces metabolic syndrome with all its complications including fatigue, obesity, diabetes, tooth decay, arterial and heart disease, cancer and dementia.
		Low in fat	'Fat is the most valuable food known to Man' – Dr John Yudkin, Founding Professor, Department of Dietetics, Queen Elizabeth College, London Increases risk of dementia ('type 3 diabetes')
		Low in fibre	Increases risk of gut cancers
		Low in micronutrients	Accelerated ageing
		No 'real' fermented foods	The consumption of live ferments extends longevity
		Alcohol	Highly toxic and addictive

		High in the major allergens – namely, gluten and dairy.	Food allergy and intolerance are estimated to cause ill health in over one third of Westerners. See our book *Sustainable Medicine*.
	Easy, convenient, cheap, quick…	…but addictive and toxic	I believe that sugar and refined carbohydrates are more dangerous to health than smoking. They are more addictive because they are still socially acceptable.
Paleo diet	No gluten grains No dairy No refined sugar Includes fermented foods		Avoids the major allergens that commonly cause irritable bowel syndrome, psychiatric conditions, migraine and headaches, asthma, eczema, arthritis and many other such inflammatory conditions. See our book *Sustainable Medicine*.
		Allows fruit, potato, non-gluten cereals and natural sugars. May be high in sugar and starch.	This can induce meta-bolic syndrome. See our book *Prevent and Cure Diabetes*.
Ketogenic diet, such as Atkins	High in fat Low in carbs High in micronutri-ents		Highly effective for reversing obesity and diabetes.
		High in dairy products…	…which are: a common cause of allergy; growth promoting (so increased risk of cancer); and a major risk factor for heart disease and osteopo-rosis.
		High in artificial sweeteners	Many, such as aspartame, are toxic, triggering headaches, depression, seizures and attention-deficit disorder, as well as cancer and birth defects. In addition, sweeten-ers maintain the sweet taste addiction.

Low-fat slimming diets		Often rely on carbs as a fuel source	The body ends up in the 'metabolic hinterland' (see Chapter 1, page 3), unable to get fuel from carbs or fat. This diet results in fatigue, foggy brain and feeling cold and depressed, which is why it is unsustainable. It requires massive determination (which I, for one, do not possess). This diet does not switch off the carbohydrate craving and does not permit fat burning except through starvation; in the long term this results in yo-yo weight swings.
		Low in fat	See above.
		High in artificial sweeteners	See above.
GAPS diet (see www. gapsdiet. com)	A good step towards a PK diet...	...but allows fruit and cheese	For some this diet will be sufficient to solve their health problems, but fruit, which it allows, is a bag of sugar and as potentially dangerous as the white stuff. The dairy products it includes are common allergens.
Vegetarian diets	High in fibre	May be low in protein	Protein is essential for tissue healing and repair
		High in carbohydrates	Metabolic syndrome is a risk – see above and also our book *Prevent and Cure Diabetes*.
		High in allergens such as dairy and gluten	Not a good diet for the allergic – at least one third of the population suffer symptoms due to food allergy or intolerance.
		May be low in micronutrients such as iron and vitamin B12	

Vegan	See above for vegetarian, plus dairy-free	See above for vegetarian with vitamin B12 being even more of an issue	
		Difficult to eat sufficient fat	
Allergy exclusion diets	Low in allergens	May be high in carbohydrates	
	Can become too restricted and calorie deficient		
The PK diet	High fat High fibre Low carb Low allergen Rich in micronutri-ents Low chemical and toxic burden Not addictive		The starting point for preventing and treating most diseases, but not all; unfortunately it does not stop me falling off my horse; it just increases the desire to ride more!
		Initial difficulties to keto-adapt (that is, switch to burning fat as the major fuel) with a difficult passage through the metabolic hinter-land. Get organised and change the habits of a lifetime! Anti-social (because few others have woken up to the benefits of it)	All these problems are solved by turning the pages of this book… read on, my friend!

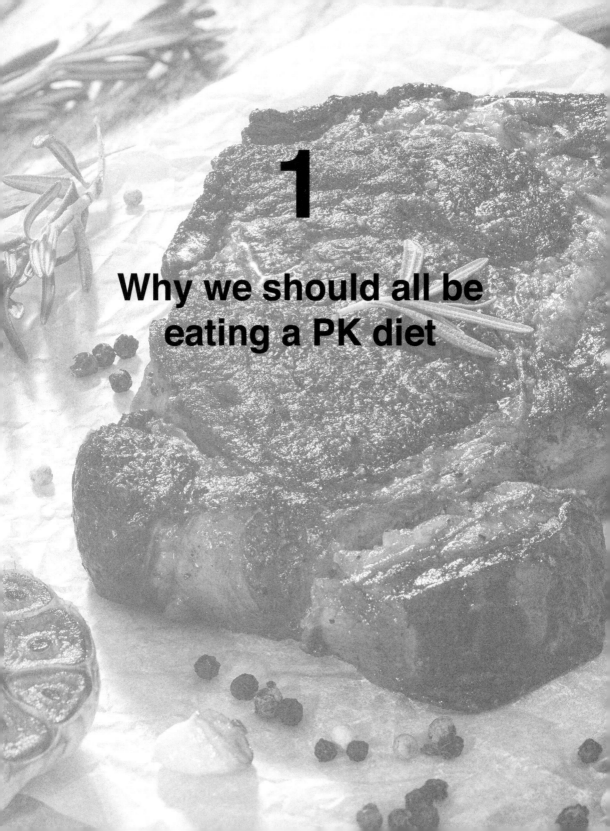

1

Why we should all be eating a PK diet

'Let food be thy medicine and medicine be thy food.'

Hippocrates, 'father of medicine', c. 460 – c. 370 BC

Humans evolved over two and half million years eating a ketogenic, paleo (PK) diet. This, as I explained in the Introduction, is a diet that:
- follows the seasons
- is pre-agricultural so excludes grain, refined carbs and dairy products
- is high in fat and vegetable fibre as alternative energy sources to sugar (respectively, ketones and short-chain fatty acids) and low in sugar and starchy carbs.

It is the diet which best suits our bowels, body and brains, as you will find if you follow the guidance in this book. If we wish to live to our full potential in terms of quality and quantity of life, this is the diet naturally selected through evolution. (At the same time we should note that evolution is served only in getting us to childbearing age. Once the 'selfish gene' of Richard Dawkins' book of that name has been passed on to the next generation, we are effectively on the evolutionary scrap heap, though we may have plenty of uses, for example looking after our grandchildren while our children go hunting and foraging.)

We should all be eating the PK diet all the time, but as we age, our bowels, bodies and brains work less efficiently and so the imperative to stick with this diet increases. Younger people can get away with less correct diets and this leads many to believe that their present diet is okay because 'that is what I have always eaten'.

'They [young people] have exalted notions, because they have not been humbled by life or learned its necessary limitations; moreover, their hopeful disposition makes them think themselves equal to great things – and that means having exalted notions. They would always rather do noble deeds than useful ones. Their lives are regulated more by moral feeling than by reasoning – all their mistakes are in the direction of doing things excessively and vehemently. They overdo everything – they love too much, hate too much, and the same with everything else.'

Aristotle, 384 – 322 BC

Or, as Oscar Wilde put it:

'Youth is wasted on the young.'

'Metabolic syndrome' is the pre-diabetic state in which blood sugar levels see-saw between too high and too low in the presence of excessively high levels of insulin. It carries many risks to health but was once a helpful tool to allow primitive man to survive winters. The idea is that when the autumn windfall of ripe fruits, seeds, nuts and root vegetables comes, the carbohydrate craving is switched on as we feast on the natural and delicious autumn harvests. This makes us fat (providing food storage and winter insulation) and lethargic (which is good for energy conservation). A high-carbohydrate diet switches on the hormonal response – primarily insulin – which inhibits fat burning (insulin lays down fat) – but also mild hypothyroidism (low thyroid hormones, so a lowered metabolic rate). Of course, when the autumn feast comes to an end, because it runs out or rots, *Homo sapiens* must switch back into normal fat-burning (ketogenic) mode.

Primitive man gained huge evolutionary advantage through being able to run on two fuels – fats and carbohydrates. Indeed, we can eat a greater variety of foods than any other mammal (bar perhaps the pig – I love pigs). This metabolic flexibility plus the first Agricultural revolution at around 10,000 BC meant that more people survived, the land could support more of us and so more people achieved child-bearing age than ever before. The population of earth sky-rocketed with this 'dual fuel effect'. However, what gets us to child-bearing age is not necessarily good for longevity. Having metabolic syndrome that is prolonged for years will dump us prematurely on the evolutionary scrap heap that I have already described.

Modern Western *Homo sapiens* lives in a state of permanent autumn with addictive carbohydrate foods constantly, conveniently and cheaply available. We are in permanent metabolic syndrome with all the short-term (fat and fatigue) and long-term (heart disease, cancer and dementia) problems associated with such (again, see our book *Prevent & Cure Diabetes*).

Getting through the 'metabolic hinterland'

The metabolic switch from burning sugar and starches to fat and fibre is difficult because it is metabolically easier to burn sugar and starch. Burning fat is less efficient and more metabolically expensive (which is why the Atkins diet (see Table 1, page xi) is so effective). There is a horrible inertia in the system which means that during the switch we have a deeply unpleasant window of time when we cannot burn carbohydrate (because we are cutting them out) and we cannot burn fat (because it takes a couple of weeks for the hormonal system to switch into fat-burning mode). What we experience in this window of time is called 'metabolic inflexibility' and the more flexible we are metabolically the shorter this period. It is so easy to give up during this time – the metabolic hinterland – and just go back to our old ways of eating cheap addictive carbohydrates. In the short term, this will give us our fix and we will 'feel better', but in the longer term, this course of action has disastrous consequences. This desire to 'take the easy route' has been an essential part of survival but now, in times of plenty, it is a damned nuisance!

The journey through this metabolic hinterland must become your personal crusade, indeed your *Pilgrim's Progress*. Craig and I have done it and can now smile smugly from a ketogenic nirvana, but at least we are cheering you on from the other side… so read on and be encouraged.

In summary, what we call the metabolic hinterland is characterised by:
- Fatigue, feeling cold, foggy brain and depression: Lack of fuel (either carbohydrates or fats) for the body to burn results in these horrible symptoms.
- Cravings: The temptation to go for instant relief of these ghastly symptoms by eating carbohydrate, such as a banana.
- But this spikes insulin.
- Worse symptoms: An hour later we again find ourselves in the metabolic hinterland with the worst of both worlds – the banana fuel has run out and the insulin spike means we cannot burn fat for some hours. Back to the fatigue, the freezer, the fog and the funk hole.
- Worse cravings: The overwhelming temptation, which subverts all else, is to eat another banana… and so it goes on, just like the drug addict.

This explains why so many people struggle initially with the PK diet. They start off by cutting down on carbohydrates instead of drastically reducing them. They drop into the metabolic hinterland and get stuck there, lethargic, foggy, cold and depressed. Instant relief is just a banana away, short-term temptation prevails and they slip back into metabolic syndrome. We must do better than Oscar Wilde:

'I can resist anything except temptation.'

Oscar Wilde, 1854–1900

Clinical applications of the PK diet

I had to work in the field of ecological medicine for 35 years, see over 20,000 patients, write three books with Craig – namely, *Sustainable Medicine, Diagnosis and Treatment of Chronic Fatigue Syndrome and Myalgic Encephalitis* and *Prevent and Cure Diabetes* – to convince myself that the PK diet was the diet we should all be eating. Since I do not ask my patients to do anything that I myself don't do (or at least have tried), I started this diet myself. I have to say that I experienced a great sense of bereavement. Was I going to miss all those foods I loved and had become used to eating? Cream, especially. But having established myself on this diet, I now know that this is what I shall be eating for the rest of my life.

As I get older, and perhaps wiser, I find myself spending more and more time discussing diet. This is the starting point for treating absolutely everything. However, it is also the most difficult thing I ask my patients to do. If I give them a list of interventions they need to make, they tend to cherry pick, choosing the easy things first. This invariably means that the diet is the last thing to change.

Diet is the first thing we could and should be addressing to restore health. The upside of this is that diet is something we can all do – the treatment is in your shopping basket and kitchen and on your plate. You don't need any physicians, pills or potions! Dietary changes are empowering – they allow us to take back control of our health. However, dietary changes are also the most difficult for all the reasons that we detail in *Prevent and Cure Diabetes*: addiction, habit and convenience. The job of this recipe book is to try to make these dietary changes much easier.

Note from Craig: Before becoming a ketogenic, I would eat at least six packets of ready-salted crisps a day. I even had a stash, and a secret stash, in case of emergencies, just like Hugh Laurie's Gregory House *and his Vicodin. I stopped all crisps on one day and have never gone back. It is not easy though – even the rustle of a crisp packet brings back memories and I have a Pavlovian response of salivation to this day!*

My job is to get patients well as quickly as possible. I used to try to be nice to my patients and pussy-foot about, trying dairy-free diets, gluten-free diets, low-carbohydrate diets, or whatever. These days I am much nastier – as I cruelly say, 'My job is to get you well, not to entertain you'. So, I start off with the toughest diet in order to get my patients well as quickly as possible. Once recovered, they can then, as

5

I call it, 'Do a deal with the devil'. Of course, we can get away with some foods on the occasional treat basis so long as we are consciously aware of what we are doing and are determined to get back on the wagon afterwards.

'Sometimes, you must be cruel to be kind.'

Old English Proverb

As I have said, this diet is paleo (no grains or dairy products) and ketogenic (low-carbohydrate, including being low in sugar, fruit sugar, grains and root vegetables). One can eat some carbohydrates, but too many and the diet fails. The aim is to fuel the body with fat and fibre, not sugar and starch. It is *not* a high-protein diet.

How you know that you have done enough to move into fat burning mode

Table 2: Symptoms, signs and disease regression associated with ketosis

Energy levels improve	See our book *Diagnosis of Chronic Fatigue Syndrome and Myalgic Encephalitis – it's mitochondria not hypochondria*
Glassy smooth teeth	Dental plaque gives teeth a rough surface. It is the biofilm behind which teeth-rotting bacteria – namely, *Streptococcus mutans* - hide. These microbes can ferment only sugar and starches. The ketogenic diet starves them out. Dental decay ceases. Halitosis is also often cured. (It may also derive from the fermenting gut and/or airway infections (chest, throat and sinus).)
Clean tongue	Tongues become dirty and discoloured because of bacterial colonies sticking to and fermenting on the tongue. Tongues should be pink and free from surface crud. (Gum disease (gingivitis) is also driven by sugar and starches.)
You may lose 1-2 kg of weight very quickly	Carbohydrates are stored in the liver and muscle as glycogen. This has an osmotic pressure – that is, it holds water. Once glycogen has been used up prior to fat burning, this water is peed out. This is one reason why endurance athletes see a rapid improvement in performance – the power/weight ratio is instantly better.
Blood sugar levels stabilise because the body is burning fat	Levels of insulin and adrenalin remain constant. (Adrenalin spikes as blood sugar levels fall in someone who is not keto-adapted – low blood sugar or 'hypoglycaemia' symptoms are largely the symptoms of adrenaline spiking (see *Prevent and Cure Diabetes*).)

You can miss a meal without getting an energy dive	One can survive on fat-burning for weeks (depending on the size of your fat store, of course). Indeed, having windows of time spent fasting stimulates new brain neurones to grow and this makes us cleverer.
You stop constantly thinking and obsessing about food	There is a constant and reliable fuel available to the body. The brain is not consumed by that next carb fix.
Urine tests (Ketostix) or blood tests show ketones are present	The ketosis (fat-burning mode) is mild, rarely above 4 pmol/l. This is not just safe but highly desirable. Please note by contrast, in the highly dangerous condition of diabetic ketoacidosis, levels are pathologically high at >20 pmol/l. Once fully keto-adapted, ketones may not show up in urine tests as the metabolism becomes more efficient.
Athletic performance improves	See above. There is a better power/weight ratio with glycogen stores depleted
Physical and mental endurance ability improves	The glycogen pantry (stored sugar in the liver and muscles) only lasts for 1,700 Kcalories (about 16 miles for marathon runners, at which point they 'hit a wall'; US athletes call this 'bonking'!). The fat pantry, even in a lean athlete, can last for up to 140,000 Kcalories.
Mental performance improves	The preferred fuel for the brain is ketones. The newborn baby runs entirely on ketones, with the brain using 60 per cent of all energy production. The ketogenic diet is the starting point for treating all brain pathologies from mental health problems and dementia to epilepsy and malignant tumours. Once keto-adapted, the blood sugar level can run as low as 1 pmol/l without symptoms arising.
You feel calmer once in established ketosis (but more anxious whilst in the metabolic hinterland)	I suspect the symptom of stress arises when the brain knows it does not have the physical, mental or emotional energy to deal with life's challenges. Being in ketosis increases the energy available in all departments. A ketogenic diet also increases levels of the calming neurotransmitter, GABA.
Gut symptoms often improve	Irritable bowel syndrome results either from food allergy (typically grains, dairy and yeast) or upper fermenting gut, often caused by SIBO (small intestine bacterial overgrowth). Reflux and bloating are typical symptoms of fermentation in the upper gut due to microbes, which should be present only in the large bowel, fermenting sugars and starches. My guess is that most bowel tumours (oesophageal, stomach and colon cancers) are driven by the fermenting gut.

Sleep quality improves – you may need fewer hours of sleep	The commonest cause of disturbed and poor quality sleep is nocturnal hypoglycaemia. Perhaps the next commonest cause is snoring due to allergy, typically to dairy products.
Any problem associated with metabolic syndrome and fermenting gut is improved – e.g. type-2 diabetes, hypertension, arthritis, irritable bladder	See our book *Prevent and Cure Diabetes*. Many conditions I suspect are driven by allergy to gut microbes. These include polymyalgia rheumatica, many arthritides (e.g. rheumatoid arthritis, ankylosing spondylitis), venous ulcers, autoimmune conditions, intrinsic asthma, psoriasis, chronic urticaria, interstitial cystitis, many psychiatric conditions, inflammatory bowel disease and nephritis. See our book *Sustainable Medicine*.
The quality of skin and mucous membranes improves	Dry skin, dry eyes, dry mouth, dry perineums (vulva and vagina) may result from low-fat diets. A high-fat diet can reverse these.
Protection from infections	The immune system, like the brain, prefers to run on fats. Infecting microbes largely run on sugar so, for example, diabetics are at much greater risk of infection. Indeed, the starting point for treating all acute and chronic infection is the PK diet. The PK diet is antifungal, antibacterial and also, interestingly, antiviral (although I have yet to work out the mechanism of this!).
Any problem associated with inflammation improves	The PK diet is anti-inflammatory.
Any problem associated with fatigue improves	The preferred fuel of mitochondria is ketones. The heart and brain run 25 per cent more efficiently burning ketones compared with sugar.

'In short, let fat be thy medicine and medicine be thy fat!'
Dr Gabriela Segura, consultant cardiologist and cardiothoracic surgeon

The future

Following the PK diet is highly protective against the diseases associated with Western lifestyles. It is also highly protective against infection. Throughout evolution, populations have been controlled by disease. This will inevitably come again in the form of a new plague, perhaps compounded by antibiotic resistance. Those people clever enough to work out that the PK diet is the one we should be doing *and* who are disciplined enough to hold it in place, will be the survivors of this plague. Natural selection and the survival of the fittest will prevail! Perhaps this provides you with an extra incentive to act now?

JUST DO IT. What follows in this book shows you how.

I am no cook, but with a little experimenting and reading I have found and developed a few recipes which abolished my sense of food-bereavement, so I no longer feel deprived. Initially, you may not have the time, energy or inclination to prepare food, so this book is organised in the following sections:

1. Meals which need no cooking or preparation – These are for people initially with no energy, time or inclination. Yes, the PK diet may be boring at first, but, as I have said, my job is to get you well not to entertain you – the rest of the book provides the entertainment. However, as you journey, you will discover that the energy, time and inclination (in that order) will follow naturally.
2. How to make PK bread (page 23). Lack of a great bread is a major source of bereavement and cause of long-term PK diet failure.
3. How to make PK 'dairy' products (page 32). As above.
4. The rest of the book – how to adapt your life and cooking to make the PK diet truly sustainable in the long term.

'Don't be afraid to take a big step if one is indicated. You can't cross a chasm in two small jumps.'

David Lloyd George, 17 January 1863 – 26 March 1945

It's important to note that this book lays down the general principles of how to eat paleo-ketogenically. It is not a recipe book, or cookbook (despite the title!), in the traditional sense of the term, although there are many delicious recipes included. In a sense this book is about a way of living. I often say to my patients that this diet is just like cricket – I can teach you the rules (or should that be laws?) of the game, but I cannot teach you how to play. Geoffrey Boycott and Sir Ian Botham both followed the laws of the game (mostly!) and both played very well (mostly) and yet they were very different players with idiosyncratic styles. So, for example, with this diet, precise amounts of each food and detailed measuring are not included. The idea is that you progress as follows:

- Follow the guidelines in Chapter 2 as to how to get into a state of ketosis (burning fat for energy).
- Initially use Ketostix (see page 137) to check that you are in ketosis. This may take some trial and error on your part to get the proportions of food that work for you. We are all so different that I simply cannot give 'one size fits all' guidance here. Craig can eat 90 grams of carbs a day and happily stay in ketosis whereas I have to stick to 30 grams of carbs or less a day. Dammit!
- Be aware that men generally move into ketosis more quickly than women, largely because female sex hormones are conducive to metabolic syndrome.
- Once you have established a state of ketosis, checked by the Ketostix, you will learn to 'recognise' when you are in this state and will 'know' when you have kicked yourself out of it too. Craig, for example, knows when he is out of ketosis because mental sharpness declines dramatically and then, once back into ketosis, he can think with clarity again – it is almost like an electric buzz in his brain. We all have our own individual signs of being in ketosis that you will come to recognise.
- At this point you will no longer need the Ketostix.

Throughout this book, I make reference to some foods by saying 'check the carbs' or suchlike. What I mean by this is that these foods are high in carbs and that you must handle (and eat!) these foods with caution. Once again, I simply cannot be prescriptive here. Appendix 3 (page 115) will give you net carb values for many 'pure' foods but as soon as there are combinations you will have to rely on labels.

Now it is time to learn the rules and develop your own style of playing the game!

(For those of you who are struggling to find your own individual style of 'playing', there is a seven-day meal plan in Appendix 5 (page 125). This may get you started but it is not recommended for long-term use as you will get bored and boredom may lead to failure. There are many exciting and delicious recipes in the pages that follow and this is how you will become a world-class paleo-ketogenic.)

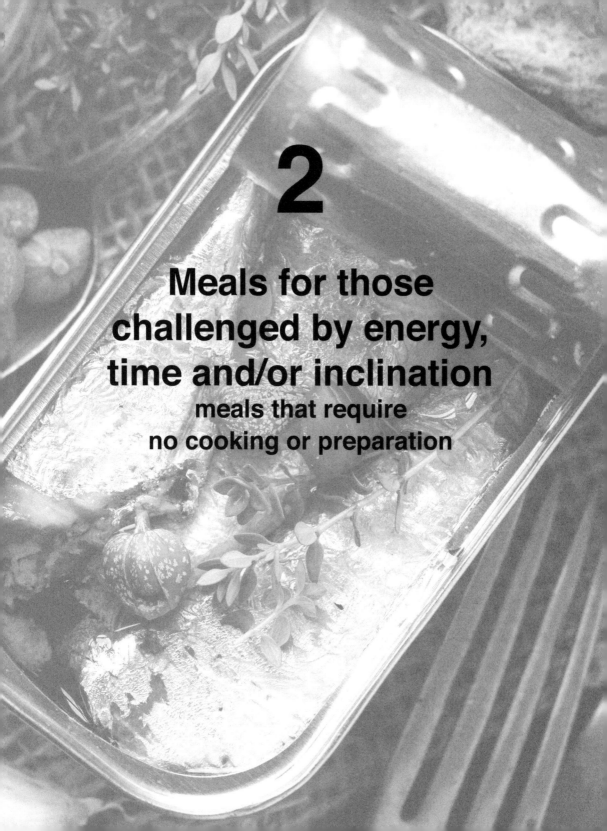

2

Meals for those challenged by energy, time and/or inclination
meals that require
no cooking or preparation

Some readers may be tempted to skip this chapter, which is primarily designed for the severely fatigued who are unable to cook meals for themselves and require carers to shop and cook for them. I would advise against doing this – there are some excellent meal ideas here, and useful websites, which will also benefit the less fatigued, and especially those who are busy and need some 'quick meal' options.

Introduction

The meal suggestions and foods listed below do not make for inexpensive eating. However, the idea of this starting phase is to get into ketosis (fat-burning mode) with minimal expenditure of time and energy. Once keto-adapted, energy levels improve so you can then move onto the recipes in subsequent chapters. The severely fatigued will need help with ordering these foods.

Initially you cannot rely simply on what you eat and how much you eat to know that you have done enough to get into ketosis. Some people can eat 100 grams of carbs per day and get there. Some have to reduce to below 30 grams (includes me – dammit!). So, use Ketostix (see Resources, page 137) to test your urine to show you are in ketosis – this is necessary because we are all different, as above. Generally, men move into ketosis more easily than women. This is because female sex hormones are conducive to metabolic syndrome. With time you will learn to recognise the 'feel' of ketosis so Ketostix will become a thing of the past.

Factors that inhibit ketosis

If you really struggle to get through the metabolic hinterland – that is to say, if after two weeks you feel terrible and cannot get into ketosis – consider the following common reasons for this:

- Alcohol is a solvent and so a sweet alcoholic drink results in a very rapid rise in blood sugar. For example, beer has a higher glycaemic index than sugar (that is, it raises blood sugar levels more quickly). Hormonal responses to blood sugar levels are proportionate to the *rate of change* rather than the absolute level (see our book *Prevent and Cure Diabetes* for more detail on this). Furthermore, alcohol stimulates insulin release directly and so a sugar-free alcoholic drink is almost as bad. Artificial sweeteners also destabilise blood sugar – see Chapter 10, page 67.

- Are you fooling yourself? Addiction makes us rationalise the irrational and deny the bleeding obvious. An insulin spike (from a moment of indiscretion, such as snaffling a bar of cheap chocolate or a bag of crisps or a biscuit, usually because 'I deserve it') will spike insulin and switch off fat burning for many hours. This means you will have a window of time of some hours when you cannot access fuel either from carbs (because the sugar spike has been pushed into fat by insulin) or from fat (because insulin blocks this). This may mean you feel awful for those hours. Knowing this is good incentive to stay on the wagon.
- A ketogenic diet is demanding of minerals; you may need extra salt (see Chapter 13: Sunshine minerals, page 93, and Appendix 4: Nutritional supplements, page 121).
- To be able to burn fat you need thyroid hormones, so get your thyroid checked. This can be easily done through the Natural Health Worldwide website (www. naturalhealthworldwide.com – see page 153).
- The Pill and HRT (hormone replacement therapy) drive metabolic syndrome and inhibit fat burning. These hormones in these medicines induce a pregnancy-like hormonal state with many of the risks associated with such – namely, high blood pressure, weight gain, type-2 diabetes, mental health problems, thrombosis and immune suppression.

Meal suggestions

Table 3 lists suggested meals that will provide healthy levels of nutrients while keeping your carb intake low. As ever, we cannot be prescriptive because your carb intake for getting into ketosis will be individual to you. However, Appendix 5 (page 125) does give a plan to get you started if necessary.

Table 3: Nutritious meals with low carbs

Meal	Foods	Notes
Breakfast	Pot of Coyo yoghurt 125 grams	Mix in ground linseed. Adjust the amount to prevent constipation. Once keto-adapted, the PK bread takes over this function
	Alpro vanilla yoghurt 200 grams or Provamel, which is also sugar-free	Fat satisfies the appetite
	Coyo chocolate yoghurt 125 grams	Ditto
Lunch and supper		

Starters	2 x avocado pears
	Large dollop mayonnaise with:
	   Slices salami, Parma ham
	   Celery stick with paté
	   Cucumber, tomato
	Sauerkraut, pickled gherkins
	Coleslaw
	Tinned vegetable low-carb soup – stir in dollop of tinned coconut milk to give it substance	

A meal in itself	Coconut paleo wraps – expensive but delicious ... use sparingly	Take care ... a single 14 gram wrap contains 3 grams of carbohydrate
Main course	Cold meat – ham, chicken, etc Tinned fish or shellfish Tinned meat Smoked mackerel fillets Tofu or quorn with pesto Washed salad – just open the package!	
Puddings	Coyo yoghurt Soya yoghurt Berries (fresh or frozen) with large dollop of Grace coconut milk	If still hungry drink the Grace coconut milk. This is by far and away the best coconut milk. Insist on the carton which for some odd reason is far superior to the tinned.

Snacks	Pork scratchings Olives 85% dark chocolate Spoonful of nut butter (eat off the spoon) Biltong	Use neem tooth picks if meat gets stuck between teeth Always count the carbs of nuts and nut butters because it is easy to overdo them (see Appendix 3, page 115).
Drinks Ad lib	Coffee with large dollop coconut cream Black tea Herbal teas Sparkling water	Caffeine has a long half-life and may disturb sleep so avoid after 2 pm.

Weekly shopping list (by Craig)

As time goes by, you will have increased energy levels and so you will be able to vary your diet and move onto the recipes in subsequent chapters. See also the useful websites on page 137 for more variety. The idea here is to keep it very simple and also to have foods that can be ordered online and delivered to your house so as to reduce energy expended on shopping expeditions.

I have included seven breakfasts, seven lunches and seven suppers below and some snacks too – there is one snack per day in this list. Regarding drinks, do concentrate on water – limit coffee and tea to a maximum of three cups a day.

For ease of shopping, I have listed the items and how to search for them on Ocado, which I have found to be the best source. Where items are not generally available from Ocado, I have included Amazon alternatives. Of course, other major supermarkets will also be able to provide most of what is needed in a 'one stop shop'. Once you have done one or two shops, things will become much easier.

If you look elsewhere, always look at the labels which detail the carbohydrate content of foods; these are very helpful. The carbohydrate values given on labels are normally total carbs which include all starches, sugars and fibre. I prefer to use net carbs (sugars and starches, with fibre excluded) on the grounds that fibre does not spike blood sugar but is fermented into short-chain fatty acids. Linseed is a good example – it is low carb because although 100 grams contains 29 grams of total carb, 27 grams are fibre and so just 2 grams are starch and sugar.

You will need to tailor these suggestions to you personally so that you get into, and remain in, ketosis. Do not take these suggested meals as guarantors of ketosis as everybody differs. Also, these are examples only and you will become bored if you rigidly eat these meals in rotation – they are examples of the 'no preparation, no cooking meals' that are suitable for getting you into ketosis.

I have presented the shopping list in two ways:

1. By meal: I have compiled the list in this way so that you can see what a daily meal plan might look like by choosing one breakfast, one lunch, one supper and a snack. There is also an 'Others' section.
2. In one combined list, showing you what the total buy will be. This list has been compiled in this way to form an easy shopping list that can be used by someone who is shopping for you, or by you or a family member ordering the items online. Where Ocado does not (generally) stock items, I have included Amazon alternatives.

1. Shopping list by meals for one week

Breakfasts for one week
- 3 x 'natural' Coyo yoghurt 125 grams
- 2 x chocolate Coyo yoghurt 125 grams
- 1 x Alpro vanilla yoghurt 500 grams (to cover two breakfasts of 200 grams with a bit left over)

Lunches for one week
Seven starters:
- Two avocados (say, 200 grams) with mayonnaise
- Large dollop mayonnaise
- Salami – just one 'stick'
- Celery stick and paté – celery (350 grams) should last two meals. Farmhouse pork paté – 100 grams in two servings of 50 grams each – lasts two meals
- Cucumber and tomato. Cucumber – should last two meals. Tomatoes – six-pack – should last two meals
- Sauerkraut – 350 grams – should last three meals
- Carrot and coconut soup – 400 grams

Seven main courses:
- Tinned ham (200 grams) – may have to make this last for two meals – 125 grams would be ideal

- Corned beef (200 grams) – may have to make this last for two meals – 125 grams would be ideal
- Tinned mackerel – in tomato sauce (125 grams)
- Tinned tuna (160 grams)
- Tinned sardines in spicy tomato (120 grams)
- Quorn with mozzarella and pesto sauce – lasts two meals (see Table 2.2 below)
- Washed salad

Occasional: Coconut paleo wraps (from Amazon only)

Seven puddings:
- Coyo natural yoghurt (125 grams)
- Coyo chocolate yoghurt (125 grams)
- Coyo berry yoghurt (125 grams)
- 50 grams blueberries from freezer with dollop of coconut cream
- 50 grams raspberries from freezer with dollop of coconut cream
- 50 grams gooseberries from freezer with dollop of coconut cream
- 50 grams strawberries from freezer with dollop of coconut cream

Suppers for one week
Same starters, mains and pudding suggestions as for lunches – mix and match.

Snacks
- Two snacks – Black Country No Nonsense Pork Scratchings one bag – twice a week
- Two snacks – One bar Green and Black's 85% dark chocolate – half a bar counts as one snack – twice a week
- One snack – one scoop of macadamia (or hazelnut) nut butter
- One snack – Olives, say 30 grams
- One snack – Biltong, say 25 grams

In addition
- Chia seeds – say 50 grams to add to yoghurts to taste, as and when
- Linseed – say 50 grams to add to yoghurts to taste, as and when – lasts longer than one week
- Coconut milk – to fill up on if you are still hungry at night – 400mls should last about one week. I prefer Grace Coconut Milk

- Coconut cream – for use with berries as a pudding – 200 grams should last about a week

Herbal teas/coffee

To suit your personal taste as none is high carb and many have health-giving properties. Tea Lyra (www.tealyra.co.uk) have an excellent range.

2. Complete combined shopping list for one week

The list in Table 4 below covers all the food items needed for all the meals listed in Table 3. Please note that some of these items will last longer than one week – go by the advice given earlier (see page 16) as to how much to eat.

Table 4: Shopping list for one week

Shopping item	Go to Ocado and search for:	If not on Ocado, go to Amazon and search for:
5 x 'natural' Coyo yoghurt (125 grams)	'CoYo Natural Yoghurt' and select size	
4 x Coyo chocolate yoghurt (125 grams)	'CoYo Chocolate Yoghurt' and select size	
2 x Coyo berry yoghurt (125 grams)	'CoYo Berry Yoghurt' and select size	
1 x Alpro vanilla yoghurt (500 grams)	'Alpro Vanilla Yoghurt' and select size	
4 x avocados (100 grams each)	'Avocados' and select size	
Mayonnaise	'Mayonnaise' and choose to your liking – 'Delouis' looks good	
Pack of six Serious Pig Snacking salami	'Salami snacking' – and choose your own if no 'Serious Pig' available – 'Rutland Charcuterie' looks good	'Serious Pig Classic Snacking Salami' (Pack of 6)
350 grams celery	'Celery sticks 350 grams'	
100 grams Farmhouse Pork Pate	'Waitrose Farmhouse Pork Paté 100 grams'	

One cucumber	'Cucumber' and select size – 'full wholegood organic' or 'Waitrose'	
Pack of six tomatoes	'6 tomatoes' –'Essential Waitrose' or 'Ocado'	
350 grams pot organic sauerkraut	'Organic Sauerkraut 350 grams'	
Carrot and coconut soup 400 grams	'Carrot and Coconut Soup'	
2 x 200 grams tinned ham	'Tinned Ham' and select size	
2 x 200 grams corned beef	'Corned Beef' and select size	
2 x 125 grams tinned mackerel in tomato sauce	'Tinned Mackerel, Tomato' and select size	
Pack of 4 X 160 grams tinned tuna	'Tinned Tuna' and select size	
2 x 120 grams tinned sardines in spicy tomato	'Tinned Sardines, Spicy' and select size	
2 wraps (240 grams) Quorn – with mozzarella and pesto sauce	'Quorn Mozzarella & Pesto Escalopes 240 grams'	
2 x washed salad in a bag	'Salad Bag' and choose to your taste	
Pack of 14 paleo coconut wraps	NO EQUIVALENT – expensive – Amazon purchase should last weeks!	'Paleo Wraps (Coconut Wraps)(14 Wraps)'
150 grams blueberries	'Blueberries' and select size	
150 grams raspberries	'Raspberries' and select size	
200 grams gooseberries	'Gooseberries' – these are 'British Cooking Gooseberries' – not always in stock – see opposite	Waitrose online stocks 'Cooks' Ingredients Gooseberries' and Sainsbury's online stocks '400gms Gooseberries'

Shopping item	Go to Ocado and search for:	If not on Ocado, go to Amazon and search for:
227 grams strawberries	'Strawberries' and select size	
'Black Country No Nonsense Pork Scratchings'	'Pork Crackling' and select your own if no 'Black Country' – 'Awfully Posh' crackling looks good!	'Black Country No Nonsense Pork Scratchings (24 Bags)'
Green and Black's 85% dark chocolate	'Green and Black's 85%' – one bar per week	
Macadamia nut butter	'Macadamia Nut butter'	
Pot olives	'Olives' and choose to taste	
Biltong	'Biltong' and choose to taste	
Chia seeds	'Chia seeds' and choose to taste	
Linseed	'Linseed' and choose to taste	
Coconut milk	'Coconut milk 400 ml' and choose to taste	'Grace Coconut Milk'. You can order 12 x 1 litre cartons in one go.
Coconut cream	'Biona creamed coconut 200 grams'	

3

PK Bread

'Give us this day our daily bread'
>   The Lord's Prayer, Matthew 6:9–13, English Standard Version, *The Bible*

For me as a child this seemed the most important part of the Lord's Prayer. I was amused to read of another child who discerned God's full name and address from listening to the Lord's Prayer by hearing 'Our Father Wichart in Heaven. Harold be thy name … lead us not into Thames Station'. A further account of a child witnessing Christian burial rites at the graveside listened to the priest signing off with '… unto the Father, unto the Son and unto the Holy Ghost' but heard '… and to the Father, and to the Son and into the hole he goes'. This still wakes me regularly at night bubbling and choking with laughter!

The single biggest reason for lapsing from the PK diet is the absence of bread. To secure the diet for life you must first make PK bread. I have searched and nothing is currently available commercially which passes muster. Loaves will become available as demand builds, but in the meantime you have to make your own bread.

If you do not have the energy to do this yourself but have any friends or family offering to help you, then top of the list must be, 'Please make my daily bread'.

PK bread consists of just linseed, sunshine salt (see Chapter 13, page 93) and water. Americans, and others, may be more familiar with linseed being referred to as flax or flaxseed or common flax. There is technically a subtle difference – flax is grown as a fibre plant that is used for linen. Linseed is grown for its seed. The flax plant is taller than linseed and is 'pulled' by hand, or nowadays by machine.

Linseed

Linseed's species is *Linum usitatissimum*, (Latin – 'the most useful linen') and it is a member of the genus *Linum*, being in the family Linaceae. The plant species is now seen only as a cultivated plant and it seems to have been domesticated only once from the (wild) species *Linum bienne* ('pale flax'). The evidence suggests that it was first domesticated for oil, rather than fibre.[1] ('*Linum usitatissimum L.* is one of eight main 'founder crops' domesticated in the Fertile Crescent about 11,000 years ago, although there is evidence of microscopic fibres from 30,000 years ago found in a cave in Georgia. It therefore originates in the crossover period between Palaeolithic and Neolithic eras. For those interested, please see 'Flax Domestication History'.[2]
The Fertile Crescent is the region in the Middle East which curves, like a quarter-moon shape, from the Persian Gulf, through modern-day southern Iraq, Syria, Lebanon, Jordan, Israel and northern Egypt and is regarded as the 'cradle of civilisation'.)

How to make a PK bread loaf in five minutes*

Please forgive the tiresome detail, but you must succeed with your first loaf because then you will be encouraged to carry on. I can now put this recipe together in five minutes (proper minutes that is – not the 'and this is what I did earlier' TV version). I have spent the last six months making a loaf almost every morning – there have been many revisions and the version below is the current recipe which I think is perfect!

Equipment needed:

- Weighing scales
- Nutribullet (or similarly effective grinding machine – do not attempt to do this with a pestle and mortar; I know – I have tried and failed)
- Mixing bowl
- A 500 gram (or one pound in weight) loaf baking tin
- Dollop of coconut oil or lard
- Paper towels

- Measuring jug
- Cup in which to weigh the linseed
- Wooden spoon
- One teaspoon of sunshine salt (or unrefined sea salt)
- Cooking oven that gets to at least 220 degrees Centigrade
- Wire rack for cooling

Table 5: Instructions for PK bread

Actions	Notes
Take 250 grams of whole linseed	You could purchase linseed in 250 gram packs and that saves weighing it. Use dark or golden linseed grains – the golden grains produce a brown loaf, the dark a black one. Do not use commercially ground linseed – the grinding is not fine enough, also it will have absorbed some water already and this stops it sticking together in the recipe. If you purchase linseed in bulk then you must weigh it really accurately in order to get the proportion of water spot on.
	No raising agent is required.

* For a slightly different version of PK bread developed by Dr Myhill's Facebook group see page 138.

Actions	Notes
Pour half the linseed into the Nutribullet/grinder together with one rounded teaspoon of PK 'Sunshine' salt (see page 93). Grind into a fine flour.	Use the flat blade to get the finest flour. Grind until the machine starts to groan and sweat with the effort! You need a really fine flour to make a good loaf. This takes about 30 seconds. The finer you can grind the flour the better it sticks together and the better the loaf. I do this in two batches of 125 grams or the blades 'hollow out' the mix so that half does not circulate and grind fully.
Pour the ground flour into a mixing bowl.	
Repeat the above with the second half of the seeds and add to the mixing bowl.	Whilst this is grinding, measure the water you need.
Add in *exactly* 270 ml water (not a typo – 270 it is). Chuck it all in at once; do not dribble it in. Stir it with a wooden spoon and keep stirring. It will thicken over the course of 30 seconds. Keep stirring until it becomes sticky and holds together in a lump.	The amount of water is critical. When it comes to cooking, I am a natural chucker in of ingredients and hope for the best. But in this case, you must measure. Initially it will look as if you have added far too much water, but keep stirring.
Use your fingers to scoop up a dollop of coconut oil or lard. Use this to grease the baking tin.	Your hands will be covered in fat which means you can pick up your sticky dough without it sticking to your hands.
Use your hands to shape the dough until it has a smooth surface. Drop it into the greased baking tin.	Spend about 30 seconds doing this. Do not be tempted to knead or fold the loaf or you introduce layers of fat which stop it sticking to itself. This helps prevent the loaf cracking as it rises and cooks (although I have to say it does not matter two hoots if it does. It just looks more professional if it does not!)
Let the loaf 'rest' for a few minutes…	…so it fully absorbs all the water and becomes an integral whole. This is not critical but allows enough time to…
…rub any excess fat into your skin, where it will be absorbed.	There is no need to wash your hands after doing this – the basis for most hand creams is coconut oil or lard. (Yes, lard. It amuses me that rendered animal fat is a major export from our local knacker man to the cosmetic industry.)

Put the loaf into the hot oven – at least 220°C (430°F) – for 60 minutes	Set a timer or you will forget – I always do! I do not think the temperature is too critical – but it must be hot enough to turn the water in the loaf into steam because this is what raises it. I cook on a wood-fired stove and the oven temperature is tricky to be precise with. That does not seem to matter so long as it is really hot. Indeed, I like the flavour of a slightly scorched crust.
Wipe out the mixing bowl with a paper towel.	This cleaning method is quick and easy. The slightly greasy surface which remains will be ideal for the next loaf. The point here is that fat cannot be fermented by bacteria or yeast and does not need washing off mixing and cooking utensils. My frying pan has not been washed for over 60 years. I know this because my mother never washed it either.
When the timer goes off, take the loaf out of the oven, tip it out and allow it to cool on a wire rack. Once cool keep it in a plastic bag in the fridge.	It lasts a week kept like this and freezes well too. It is best used sliced thinly with a narrow-bladed serrated knife.

Taste

At my first writing of this chapter I stated: 'Do not expect this bread to taste and perform exactly like a conventional wheat-based loaf.' However, my PK bread recipe has evolved so much in the six months of experimentation that many of my greatest critics (one of whom has been me) have been won over. The resultant loaf, made with golden linseed, looks exactly like a small brown Hovis.

The name Hovis was coined in 1890 by London student Herbert Grime in a national competition set by S. Fitton & Sons Ltd to find a trading name for their patent flour which was rich in wheat-germ. Grime won £25 when he coined the word from the Latin phrase hominis vis *– 'the strength of man'. The company became the Hovis Bread Flour Company Limited in 1898.*

Even if the loaf does not initially taste good to you, keep at it. Taste is acquired. A dear friend and colleague – namely, the late Dr Alan Franklin, consultant paediatrician at Chelmsford, UK – ran a trial with his allergic child patients. They, too, had to avoid grains and dairy. With their agreement, they ate a portion of their least favourite food daily. This included foods that kids often dislike, such as Brussels sprouts, mushrooms and avocado pears. No child had to eat the food more than 14 times (that is, two weeks) before coming to like it.

Historical note: Brussels sprouts seem to have had a mysterious history. Some sources indicate that they were eaten in classical times, but the evidence is not conclusive. English food writer Jane Grigson states that they are first mentioned in the city of Brussels market regulations in 1213, thus giving rise to their name. Mention of Brussels sprouts certainly appears about 200 years later on the menus of Burgundian wedding feasts held at the court of Lille.

The point here is, we are not born with taste preferences, we acquire them. Primitive man, pottering through the jungle, would have tried new foods with great suspicion and reluctance. However, if he was not poisoned, but rather nourished by that food, then he would have eaten more and more of it and eventually would have come to like it. By way of association of sensation, taste and satiety, he would have progressed to actively seeking out that food. In the long term he came to farm and harvest it.

The above scenario reflects my personal journey with linseed bread. I initially viewed my dark brown brick with distaste and suspicion. I forced it down out of a sense of loyalty to the diet. However, as I perfected the above recipe I came to look forward to, and love, it. It has character, texture and taste. It forms part of every breakfast and supper. My breakfast invariably includes PK fried bread – that is, linseed bread fried in coconut oil or lard. My suppers often start with PK toast.

Linseed is particularly helpful because the PK diet can make one constipated. The high fibre content of linseed mitigates this. This fibre is fermented in the large bowel to produce short-chain fatty acids. These nourish the lining of the large bowel directly and this is highly protective against bowel cancer. Fermentation of vegetable fibre also produces hydrogen and methane. These gases make you fart, but they are odourless. Put a match to them and they will explode, not that I recommend this for diagnostic purposes! If your farts smell offensively then that is due to poor digestion of foods – the fermentation of protein produces the disgusting pong of hydrogen sulphide. The constituents of smelly farts are carcinogenic – in other words, you can determine the potential health of your large bowel by smell.

Indeed, Professor Gibson, a food microbiologist from the University of Reading, divides people into 'inflammables' and 'smellies' – the inflammables (hydrogen and methane) have normal gut fermentation and the smellies (hydrogen sulphide) do not.

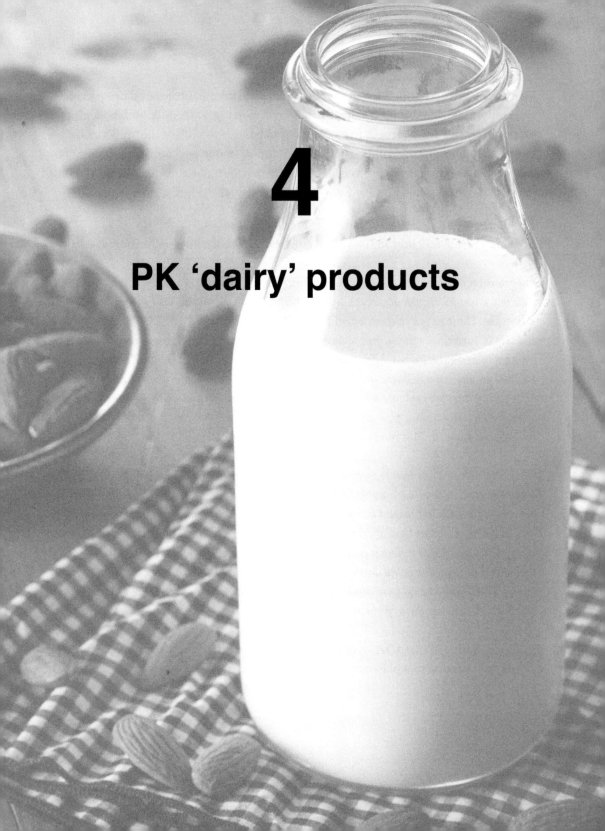

4

PK 'dairy' products

Many passages and quotations from bygone days extol the virtues of dairy products, especially milk. Exodus 33.3 talks of the 'land flowing with milk and honey' as a promised land. Lady Macbeth fears that her husband is too full of the 'milk of human kindness', again placing 'milk' as a positive notion in our psyche. So, the belief that dairy products are healthy for us is deeply entrenched in our culture. It is well then to pause and consider this Received Wisdom and consider the facts.

> *'We do not receive wisdom; we must discover it for ourselves.'*
> Marcel Proust, 10 July 1871 – 18 November 1922, French novelist, critic and essayist

But before we do this, let us not forget Cleopatra, who had other uses for milk! It is often quoted, with much historical evidence, that Cleopatra bathed in sour donkey's milk to improve the look of her skin. The logic goes that when milk sours, lactose is converted by bacteria into lactic acid and this in turn causes the surface layer of the skin to peel off, leaving new, smoother, blemish-free skin underneath. Indeed, lactic acid is an example of an alpha-hydroxy acid, and such acids are used in modern-day cosmetics for 'wrinkle-free skin' – so this story is plausible. But this is an early example of symptom suppression – I prefer more natural and sustainable methods of obtaining healthy skin, from the inside out – please see our book Sustainable Medicine – whistle blowing on 21st medical practice *for much more detail on this.*

However, there is a less well recognised use for which Cleopatra utilised milk; the great Queen is remembered as what we may call a toxicologist these days. She first started administering her poisons in wine but when that method became too well known and suspected, she turned to milk as her preferred method of delivery. Cleopatra was very methodical. She conducted many experiments and tested different poisons to see the effects, the lethality, and the correct dosage that would be needed to cause death, along with the amount of suffering caused by the various toxins. These experiments were carried out on men (her chosen target) and often Mark Antony was forced to witness them, perhaps as a warning.

So, with that in mind, let us return to why it is that dairy products, even when not mixed with Cleopatra's poisons, are so dangerous to us.

Why dairy products from the cow, the goat and the sheep are so dangerous to health

Dairy products have created numerous health problems in Westerners over the centuries for the reasons I will now describe.

Dairy products are major allergens

Dairy products cause allergy reactions in, I estimate, at least 20 per cent of the population. The allergen (the protein in milk, namely 'casein') remains the same throughout our lives but the target organ changes. Newborn babies may suffer projectile vomiting due to the pyloric stenosis triggered by milk protein. Even if mum is breast-feeding, this tough protein will get into the breast-milk if she is consuming it. Three-month colic is typical of dairy allergy. Thereafter, the target organ changes – next we see toddler diarrhoea. The tot may grow out of this problem but then becomes catarrhal, with snotty nose, snoring, cough and recurrent upper respiratory tract infections, including otitis media, tonsillitis, sinusitis and bronchitis. Asthma may be diagnosed and inhalers prescribed.

Later on in life, dairy allergy manifests with snoring, migraine, irritable bowel syndrome, depression and arthritis. I get a painful hip if I eat dairy products – as a child I was told I had 'growing pains' – what a joke! Indeed, I used to chat away with the late Dr Honor Anthony, Consultant Allergist.[1] She maintained that nearly all cases of arthritis were caused by allergy. At the time I dismissed this notion; I now know she was absolutely spot on. If arthritis is not from allergy to foods, then it probably results from allergy to microbes spilling over into the bloodstream from the fermenting gut. (This is called bacterial translocation.)

In the long term, chronic undiagnosed allergy often results in fatigue. I see many patients with chronic fatigue syndrome. A particularly common progression is the undiagnosed dairy-allergic child picking up recurrent infections, especially tonsillitis, then getting glandular fever and switching into a post-viral chronic fatigue syndrome. (See our book *Diagnosis and Treatment of Chronic Fatigue Syndrome and Myalgic Encephalitis – it's mitochondria, not hypochondria,* Second edition.)

Lactose intolerance

Lactose intolerance results from the lack of the enzyme (lactase) to digest milk sugar (lactose). It occurs in 5 per cent of Northern Europeans and 90 per cent of Africans and Asians. If lactose cannot be digested, it gets fermented in the gut by microbes to produce some, or all, of the symptoms of upper fermenting gut, such as bloating, pain, reflux, nausea, indigestion and diarrhoea. Please see our book *Sustainable Medicine – whistle blowing on 21st medical practice* for much more detail on this. Many cultures, such as those in the Near and Far East, do not drink fresh milk or use cream for this reason. They can only digest fermented milks or ghee.

(For those who are interested in learning more about this topic, there is an interesting webpage on ProCon.org, complete with links to studies, entitled 'Lactose Intolerance by Ethnicity and Region'.[2])

Dairy products are growth promoters

Milk has evolved over millions of years as the perfect nutrition for the mammalian baby. These babies are highly dependent on good maternal care for their survival. They need to grow and become fit and strong very quickly so that they can escape predators. This would be especially true of the ancestors of our modern cows, goats and sheep. Once born, there was little their mothers could do to protect them. Within a few hours of birth, they had, at least, to be able to keep up with the herd. Think of those wildlife programmes, with baby wildebeest being chased by carnivores. Milk was and still is full of growth promoters. Those calves, kids and lambs grew – and still grow – very quickly.

Human children fed dairy products also grow quickly. It is entirely natural that they suckle human breast-milk, but entirely unnatural that they consume the milk of other mammals. When challenged by the question, 'Are dairy products not natural foods?' a long-standing advocate of paleo diets, Dr Loran Cobain, replied: 'Have you ever tried milking a wild bison?'

We now have a generation of youngsters who are taller and fatter than ever before. Of course, carbohydrates in the form of sugar and refined starches further contribute to height and weight. Being tall and fat are both known risk factors for getting cancer. Indeed, the first positive nutritional step for preventing and treating cancer is to cut out all dairy products, sugars and carbs.

A research project called 'the Million Women Study' concluded that: 'Cancer incidence increases with increasing adult height for most cancer sites. The relation between height and total cancer RR [relative risk] is similar in different populations.'[3]

Research has shown that we all produce about 10,000 DNA mutations every second. Some will be early cancers. The immune system is well able to identify these rogue cells and kill them off before they cause problems. But if they grow too quickly, driven by dairy products and carbohydrates, they overwhelm the immune system's ability to cope with them and so tumours develop. As we age, the imperative to avoid all dairy products increases.

Dairy products increase the risk of autoimmunity

We are currently seeing epidemics of autoimmunity, with one in 20 of the population now affected. Of particular concern is the rise in type-1 diabetes in children. The three known major risk factors for this are vaccination, vitamin D deficiency and consumption of dairy products. The mechanism of this is probably that circulating antibodies against cow's milk protein cross react with part of the self, in the case of type-1 diabetes, with the Islets of Langerhan – the insulin-producing cells – in the pancreas.

There are numerous studies linking the consumption of dairy products with type-1 diabetes. The study by Gerstein (1994), 'Cow's milk exposure and type-1 diabetes mellitus. A critical overview of the clinical literature,' concluded that: 'Early cow's milk exposure may be an important determinant of subsequent type-1 diabetes and may increase the risk approximately 1.5 times.'[4]

Many of the studies on which this overview study was based, were much more direct in their conclusions. Virtanen et al (1993), in their study, 'Early introduction of dairy products associated with increased risk of IDDM [insulin-dependent diabetes mellitus, meaning type-1 diabetes here] in Finnish children', concluded that: 'This is the first observational study to show that early introduction of dairy products is independently associated with an increased risk of IDDM. Adjustment for mother's education and age, child's birth order, or birth weight did not affect the results.'[5]

Dairy products increase the risk of osteoporosis

When I suggest people stop consuming dairy the immediate riposte is, 'What about my calcium?' and then 'Will I not get osteoporosis?' In fact, calcium is a side issue – there is plenty of calcium (and more important than calcium, magnesium) in PK foods – but two greater issues that are often forgotten are:

1. How well is calcium (and magnesium) absorbed? and
2. Where is it deposited in the body?

Vitamin D is the key. Vitamin D greatly enhances the absorption of calcium (and magnesium) but, as importantly, stimulates its deposition in bone. Indeed, magnesium is more important than calcium in the prevention and treatment of osteoporosis. The proportion of calcium to magnesium in dairy products is 10:1 but our physiological requirements are 2:1. Since calcium and magnesium compete for absorption, dairy products induce a magnesium deficiency. It may be that this is the mechanism by which dairy products increase the risk of osteoporosis.

Dairy products are a risk factor for heart disease

A good friend and colleague, Dr David Freed, produced a paper called 'The cow and the coronary'. It concluded that the non-fat aspects of milk (the poor calcium/magnesium ratio together with lactose and milk factor antibodies) strongly correlated with deaths from heart disease. Milk factor antibodies bind to blood platelets (the cells that work to stop bleeding), resulting in sticky blood.[6]

Conclusion: do not eat dairy products but butter may be OK

If you suffer no symptoms or diseases and are otherwise completely well, then I do permit just one dairy product – that is butter. Dairy fat is the safest part of dairy products, and better than butter is ghee. This is butter that has been warmed so the dangerous cow's milk protein floats to the top and is scraped off as a white scum, leaving clear yellow pure fat behind.

PK dairy products

Giving up dairy products was, for me, a bereavement. I so loved cream! However, the alternatives in Table 6 have changed all that and I now enjoy PK alternatives. This is largely because coconut milk and palm oil have almost identical medium-chain fats to dairy products. These medium-chain fats (see Appendix 1, page 109) impart a similarly smooth texture, which means that we can make excellent dairy alternatives with them. These can be used interchangeably with dairy in the following ways:

Table 6: PK dairy alternatives

PK milk	Soya milk, coconut milk and other nut milks	Choose those that are non-GM (not genetically modified) and free from sweeteners.
PK single cream	Grace coconut milk	Comprised solely of coconut milk and water, it has a fabulous creamy texture and is an absolute essential for the PK diet. Note: the carton form is far superior to the tinned form – dunno why.
PK double cream	Grace coconut milk blended with coconut oil using sunflower lecithin – see page 34	
PK clotted cream	As above – but use more coconut oil	
PK yoghurt	Coyo	Choose the plain yoghurt. The flavoured varieties have added fruit or sugar. See recipe on page 34.
PK butter	'Crisco butter-flavour all-vegetable shortening' or 'Tiano organic exquisite 3-coconut spreadable'.	The problem with margarines is that they contain hydrogenated fats which will be partly comprised of trans fats (see Appendix 1, page 107). The butter alternatives listed here are free of trans fats.
PK cheese	The vegan cheeses are not quite the same as dairy cheeses but make an acceptable substitute: e.g. Vegusto cheese. (See www.buteisland.com for a range of excellent vegan cheeses).	A bit pricey so I use them sparingly – they do contain yeast so beware if you are allergic to yeast. Do check the carb content.
PK ice cream	An ultra-quick version is simply to pour Grace coconut milk over frozen berries and put this in deep freeze for a few minutes.	Avoid the dairy-free commercial ice creams which are high in sugar. See recipe on page 35.
PK chocolate	95 or 100 per cent dark chocolate	A bar of this lasts me several days. This tells me I am not addicted to it. Most people are addicted to the sugar and dairy content of chocolate. I know this from my own experience – a bar of 'normal', less than 85 per cent coco solids chocolate I cannot ignore!
PK coconut chocolate	See recipe on page 35	Easy to make, inexpensive and satisfying.

Table 7: PK 'dairy' recipes

	Ingredients	Actions
PK double cream	Grace coconut milk 83%: coconut oil 17% plus ½ teaspoon lecithin per 500 ml (that is, 500 ml Grace coconut milk plus 100 ml coconut oil plus ½ teaspoon lecithin)	Pour the milk and lecithin into your Nutribullet or equivalent. Warm up the oil so it pours and add to the milk. Whizz up for a few seconds. Put it in the fridge and it sets to double-cream consistency.
PK clotted cream	As above but use coconut oil 40% (that is, 300 ml Grace coconut milk plus 200 ml coconut oil plus ½ teaspoon of lecithin)	As above
PK yoghurt	Grow kefir on soya milk as detailed in Chapter 12 (page 87). Pour off excess whey then add coconut oil in the proportion 1:4 plus ½ teaspoon lecithin per 500 ml	Pour the soya (or nut) milk kefir and lecithin into the Nutribullet or equivalent. Warm up the oil so it pours and add to the milk. Whizz up for a few seconds. Put in the fridge and it sets to double-cream consistency
PK ice cream (quick version)	Cup of Grace coconut milk Lecithin, ¼ teaspoon Frozen berries – not more than a handful or it clogs up in the machine	Make this in small batches, otherwise it freezes solid and will not mix. Pour coconut milk and lecithin into the Nutribullet (or equivalent). Add the berries and immediately whizz it all up before it freezes. It should turn into a slush. Pour into a small container and freeze. If I want a large amount, I do this in several small batches – a film of coconut milk on the inside helps to prevent the mixture setting solid in the Nutribullet. (I have done it wrong lots of time by being greedy and doing too big a batch at once!) You will too, but again, as Marcel Proust said, 'We must discover it for ourselves.')

PK ice cream (long version)	Ingredients as above, but sieve out the skins and pips and put the slush into an ice cream maker. This stirs the mix constantly, so preventing ice crystals forming. This imparts that wonderful silky smooth texture.	I rarely make this because the above version is so quick, so easy and so good, with minimal washing up *and* contains all the goodness of the berry skins. I told you I was lazy!
PK coconut chocolate	Pour a whole 460 gram pot of coconut oil into a pan and warm. For mild chocolate, add the same volume of pure cocoa powder (or 1 x 125 gram pot of Green and Blacks cocoa powder). For dark choc, add twice the amount (i.e. 2 x 125 pots of Green and Blacks cocoa powder).	Mix together. Pour into ice cube containers and put in the deep freeze. Eat this PK chocolate direct from the deep freeze. It melts in the mouth just like chocolate. Coconut oil has a lower melting point than chocolate fat – it will run off the table if served at room temperature. You can of course make this using pure coco butter, but this is rather expensive.

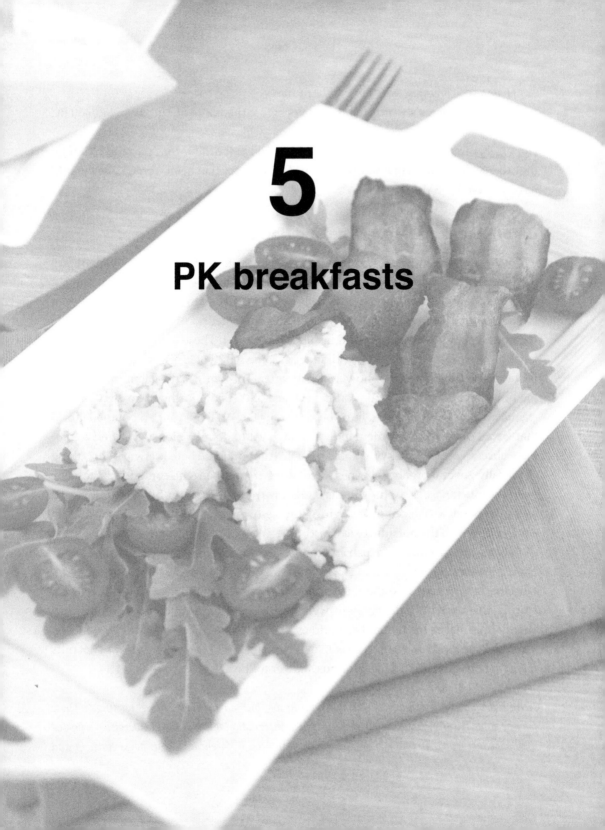

5
PK breakfasts

'Have a good breakfast men, for we dine in Hades!'
  King Leonidas's words to his soldiers before the Battle of Thermopylae, 480 BC

Hopefully things will not end the same way for us as it did for the Spartans, although they did achieve a kind of immortality … (Maybe if they had been women, they would have survived! – SM)

Before breakfast – exercise and detox

On rising, breakfast does not have to be first thing you do. Indeed, many cannot face the prospect of a substantial meal so immediately. If time permits (and see below), it is best to rise and do something physically active, sufficient to make you hot and even sweaty. Getting hot and sweaty is an excellent way to get rid of pesticide and volatile organic compounds which are held in subcutaneous fat. These 'boil off' onto the lipid layer on the surface of the skin (and, indeed, some will 'volatise' into the air). As important as getting hot is the shower or bath after. This washes the chemicals off from the now contaminated oily film on the surface of the skin. Without washing off, the chemicals simply diffuse back into subcutaneous fat. We live in such a polluted world that we all carry a toxic burden. Indeed, I have yet to do a fat biopsy and find a complete absence of pesticides or volatile organic compounds. There is always something – typically, several organochlorines, dichlorobenzenes, benzene compounds, toluene and other such nasties. Getting hot is a great way of keeping our body chemical load as low as possible. We can never reduce it to zero; the best that can be achieved is an equilibrium with the outside toxic world.

My morning routine is to rush around my small-holding, with my Patterdale terrier Nancy leading the way, feeding pigs, horses and chickens, mucking out the barn, wheelbarrowing logs into the kitchen and perhaps digging or weeding the garden. During this exercise I deliberately wear too many clothes and purposefully rush about – this makes me hot and sometimes sweaty. Cripes, I can feel Mother wincing: 'Darling,' she used to say, 'Pigs sweat, men perspire but ladies merely glow.' That puts me in the pig category. Then a glorious shower follows.

Note from Craig: *My mother used that saying too, but substituted 'horses' for 'pigs'. There may be some truth in it too – scientists at Osaka International and Kobe Universities reported that men lost twice as much moisture per square inch of forehead, chest, back, forearm and*

thigh as did women. The study included 20 women and 17 men, roughly half of whom were fit,
cycling continuously at various intensities for an hour in a room heated to 30°C.[1, 2]

My patients with CFS/ME cannot exercise. If they could, then, by definition, they would not have chronic fatigue syndrome. Exercise simply and quickly makes them much worse. However, to sauna is an equally good alternative. I know this because I have collected the results of tests of toxicity before and after sauna-ing regimes and the toxic load comes down reliably well. A rough rule of thumb is that 50 saunas halve the body's load. Traditional saunas are not tolerated by CFS sufferers because they cannot tolerate the heat. Far-infrared (FIR) saunas work as well because they just heat the subcutaneous flesh without increasing core temperature.

Readers must forgive me for this digression – but toxic stress is such a dangerous part of modern Western life and, I believe, presents a serious threat to the survival of humanity. Partly symptomatic of this is that one in seven couples are now sub-fertile and often require assisted conception. Sperm counts are falling with the percentage of abnormal results rising rapidly. Worse, serious congenital malformations (birth defects) are increasing and now afflict 3 per cent of babies.

These simple exercise and detox measures will greatly help to mitigate the problem until the politicians find a sustainable global solution to over-population and the pollution which invariably accompanies it.

The PK diet is good for sleep so you can rise earlier

The commonest cause of disturbed sleep is low blood sugar at night. Quality of sleep is improved on a PK diet as you are able to burn fat and fibre as alternative energy sources. This means you can rise sooner, which allows more time to get some sweaty work done before breakfast.

The importance of a good breakfast

Breakfast literally means to break the fast. One of the major benefits of the PK diet is that we no longer need to eat three times a day because our fat pantry (as opposed to our starch/glycogen pantry) can easily sustain us for many hours. I was blown away by a study by the Californian neurologist, Professor Dale Bredersen. He took 10 patients with Alzheimer's disease and cured nine out of 10 them with a PK diet plus other simple nutritional interventions. (The one failure was a lady who could not stick to the diet.) A feature of his regime was that the daily ration of food had to be eaten within a 10-hour window of time – that is, 14 hours of the day had to be fasting.[3]

The health benefits of fasting

Benefits for the brain

Fasting delivers a profound stimulus to the brain to create new connections, perhaps because during this time the body has to run on ketones from fats and the brain loves to run on ketones. Indeed, the newborn baby runs her metabolism entirely on fats, with the brain consuming 60 per cent of all energy generated in her body. During this time, her brain is growing and creating two million new synaptic connections every second. Even mature adults continue to make one million new connections every second. Fasting and ketosis accelerate this process. This makes perfect biological sense. During times of famine we switched into ketosis. Being in this state made us smarter. It improves our ability to communicate with each other, plan ahead, make tools for hunting, train our hounds and horses. This all happened much faster on a PK diet during fasting. Indeed, we still use fasting in modern times to sharpen our wits and brains for religious ceremonies.

A good breakfast means lunch is unnecessary. This is a huge saving of time and energy in the middle of the day when we are busiest. If you can't manage without lunch, then you are not doing the diet properly. The business of digesting lunch requires energy – I have heard so many people comment that their afternoons are more productive mentally and physically if they do not eat lunch. I use that extra window of time to nap for 30 minutes.

Benefits for the teeth, gums and gut

What rots our teeth are carbohydrates in the mouth, especially sugars. These are fermented by bacteria, namely *Streptococous mutans*, and the acidic products of fermentation dissolve teeth and rot gums. Saliva has wonderful antimicrobial properties to keep the mouth clean. As any vet will testify, a licked wound is a clean wound. The health of the mouth directly reflects the risk of heart disease and cancer, with tooth decay and gingivitis being major risk markers for both (I am not sure yet if this is a causal or a casual association). Saliva is most effective when the mouth is empty – our modern habit of snacking is very bad for oral health.

A very similar problem may occur in the upper gut. If we overeat, we overwhelm our ability to digest, and this means that carbohydrates, especially sugars, are fermented instead. Numbers of fermenting microbes build up and play havoc with gut function. I suspect this, together with allergy to foods, is the major cause of reflux oesophagitis, irritable bowel syndrome, stomach ulcers and inflammatory bowel disease. I suspect the fermenting mouth and fermenting gut are driving our current epidemics of cancer of the mouth, oesophagus, stomach and colon.

Fermentation in the lower gut – the large bowel or colon – is normal. Here we expect to harbour trillions of friendly microbes which ferment vegetable fibre into a useful fuel source – namely, short-chain fatty acids (that is, more fats). These nourish the lining of the gut directly. They also ferment to produce useful vitamins and even neurotransmitters which have calming effects on us. These friendly microbes help to program the immune system and are highly protective against infection (for more detail see our book *Sustainable Medicine*).

The bottom line is that the PK diet is the starting point for allowing us to live to our full potential as well as preventing and treating most, if not all, diseases.

Breakfast is the most important meal of the day

Breakfast is the most important meal of the day but also the one we least want to spend physical and mental energy on. Get organised. For this reason, most people have the same breakfast each day which they can make without thinking. This frees the active brain to focus on the day ahead.

> *'When you wake up in the morning, Pooh,' said Piglet at last, 'what's the first thing you say to yourself?'*
>
> *'What's for breakfast?' said Pooh. 'What do you say, Piglet?'*
>
> *'I say, I wonder what's going to happen exciting today?' said Piglet.*
>
> *Pooh nodded thoughtfully. 'It's the same thing,' he said.*
>
> AA Milne, 18 January 1882 – 31 January 1956, *Winnie-the-Pooh*

Table 7: Cooked breakfast with minimal time and effort

Take these foods:	Use the oven. Take an oven tray with a metal rack above.	
Meat: bacon, burgers, belly pork, sausage, black pudding etc	Place on top of the wire rack with strips of leaf fat or dripping.	This leaves delicious crunchy scratchings as the fat runs away.
PK bread, mushrooms, leftover green vegetables, onions, tomato, pepper or whatever	Under the rack place your PK bread and PK vegetables.	The fat runs from upstairs to downstairs so the PK bread and vegetables soak it up and cook.
	Put it all in the oven at 200°C (392°F). Set the timer for 15 minutes.	This allows you to get on with other jobs but not burn your breakfast.
	When the timer goes off, crack an egg or two into the downstairs veggie tray – the heat of the tray will cook it. Tip onto a plate and tuck in.	Do not wash out the oven tray. Leave any fat in it for the next day. Indeed, it is my opinion that fat left like this at room temperature for 24 hours is far safer than washing up and risking traces of washing-up liquid. Detergent is highly toxic to the body.

If you cannot face a full cooked breakfast...

I acknowledge that some people can't face a full cooked breakfast, though my experience is that given enough practice not only can you, but it becomes a highly desirable part of the day. The suggestions that follow sometimes require (some) cooking and sometimes little or none, but they are all designed to be less 'heavy' on the stomach, until you are ready for the Full Monty, as above.

Historical note: *The origins of the phrase 'the Full Monty' are not known for certain, but, interestingly, one possibility is the enormous breakfasts eaten by Field Marshal Montgomery (see Wikipedia).*

Suggestion 1

Several slices of PK toast (page 21) with PK butter (page 33), or fried PK bread, with:

- 2-3 boiled eggs
- Smoked fish, tinned fish, tinned cod's roe
- Paté or rillette
- Nut butter
- Vegan cheese (check the carb content of this) and tomato
- Coyo yoghurt

Suggestion 2 – PK porridge or PK muesli

The only grain which is sufficiently low-carb for this purpose is linseed.

PK porridge:

- 1 cup of ground linseed
- 4 cups of Grace coconut milk
- Cook in pan for 30-60 seconds until it thickens.
- Serve – add in berries and/or cinnamon to taste.

PK muesli:

- 1 cup of ground linseed
- 4 cups of Grace coconut milk
- Allow to stand for a few minutes for the linseed to absorb the coconut milk
- Add a large dollop of coconut or soya yoghurt.
- Add in nuts, seeds and berries to taste.

(See Appendix 3, page 115, for suggestions and carb content.)

The point with these options is that with a high proportion of linseed it is hard to overdo the nuts and seeds, which do have a higher carb percentage. So many commercial so-called ketogenic mueslis or porridges use oats, coconut, quinoa or chia as their base, but there is little hope of getting into ketosis using these grains and seeds – indeed, it would be too easy to use up one's carb allowance for the day with this one meal. Furthermore, linseed and coconut milk achieve the real aim of eating sufficient fat and fibre to satisfy the appetite and to fuel you through the day.

Suggestion 3 – Smoothies

The key to a ketogenic smoothie is to ensure high fat and fibre content, but low sugar and starch. The oily basis of the smoothie should be avocado, coconut oil or, indeed, any nut, seed or vegetable oil. A teaspoon of sunflower lecithin ensures the oil and water components are well blended to afford a wonderful silky smooth texture.

Possibly add in soya or coconut yoghurt or Grace coconut milk.

Choose salad and veg *ad lib* from the 'green list' in Appendix 3 (page 117); add others from the 'amber list', but weigh them.

Craig's all-time favourite breakfasts

- Cook asparagus in PK butter topped with ham and PK cheese
- Scrambled eggs with PK butter and smoked salmon (Craig's all-time favourite)
- Plus, see the 'no preparation' breakfasts in Chapter 2 (page 42).

The key is to keep the fat content as high as you can – try your own ideas based on these examples and add in what you fancy, always with an eye on PK butter, cream and cheese.

Shakespeare provides us with only one breakfast recipe:

'Eight wild boars roasted whole at breakfast, but twelve persons there.'

Antony and Cleopatra Act 2, Scene 1, William Shakespeare,
26 April 1564 (baptised) – 23 April 1616

6

PK starters

The origin of the 'starter' goes back a long way. Wealthy Romans generally had two main courses and before these courses they were served with small amounts of fish, vegetables, olives and even stuffed dormice – the usual stuffing was minced pork, pepper and pine kernels. These starters were known, most often, as *gustatio*.

Once you are fully keto-adapted and eating just two meals a day, you may find you need to add in a starter in order to get sufficient calories on board.

'Please, sir, I want some more.'
>Oliver, *Oliver Twist*, Charles Dickens, 7 February 1812 – 9 June 1870

'Of course, tuck in!'
>Dr Sarah Myhill (1958–2058, falls from horse permitting)

The following ideas are listed in order of ease – that is, those that require little time, energy or inclination come first.

- **Bowl of sauerkraut** - This is my favourite starter – indeed, the benefits to digestion determine this should be eaten as a starter (see Chapter 12 on fermented foods, page 83).
- **PK bread** or toast is delicious:
  - ◊ dipped in oils such as olive oil, hemp oil, rape seed oil. (This is another favourite but makes a mess of my shirt as I throw oil down the front of it – neither I nor the shirt mind too much but the person sitting opposite may. The dog is awfully pleased!)
  - ◊ with dripping and a generous pinch of sunshine salt (page 93) and pepper
  - ◊ with palm oil or coconut oil
  - ◊ dipped in PK yoghurt with garlic
  - ◊ with nut butters
  - ◊ with seed butters, such as tahini
  - ◊ with PK cheese and tomato
- **PK bread** or toast and PK butter (or PK garlic butter) makes an excellent starter with:
  - ◊ anchovies (my favourite – the oil in anchovy is particularly desirable to the brain, being rich in the omega-3 fatty acid EPA (eicosapentaenoic acid)).
  - ◊ paté – there are many excellent patés which can be purchased

- ◊ salami
- ◊ smoked fish
- ◊ tinned cod's roe
- ◊ tinned fish, crab, shellfish (mussels, cockles, whelks and winkles) with samphire
- ◊ sun-dried tomatoes
- ◊ herb spreads, such as pesto
- ◊ hummus
- ◊ olive paté
- ◊ asparagus
- ◊ mushrooms fried in lard or PK butter
- ◊ rillette (see how to make it and lard and dripping, Chapter 9, page 65)
- **French dressing or mayonnaise** (Chapter 8, page 59) with:
  - ◊ avocado
  - ◊ salad sticks, such as raw carrot, celery, fennel, beetroot, cucumber, peppers
  - ◊ pickled cucumber
  - ◊ coleslaw – finely cut, raw or grated cabbage, carrot, fennel and celery
    - * with added nuts and seeds
    - * with added shellfish, such as tinned prawns, mussels, cockles
    - * with added anchovies
- **PK soup** – If you are a particular lover of soup, you may consider purchasing a soup maker. These are brilliant. You simply chuck in all the ingredients and it chops, cooks and blends so that you have a fabulous soup 20 minutes later. *Note from Craig: Sarah bought me a soup maker. It is so easy that even I can use it. There is virtually no effort required.*

  The basic recipe is:
  - ◊ PK stock from your stock pot (see 'Bone broth', Chapter 7, page 50)
  - ◊ vegetables – whatever is in the garden, pantry, deep freeze or delivered veggie box (see Appendix 3, page 115, for the carb values of PK vegetables). My favourite vegetables would be onion, leek (remember always to include the green leaves – the whole of the leek is edible), tomatoes, celery and carrot.
  - ◊ herbs and spices that you like (for me this is garlic, black pepper, ginger).
  - ◊ Once the soup is cooked and has cooled a little, stir in a large dollop of coconut milk (or other oil, such as hemp oil) if you wish for a creamier result.

- **PK gazpacho** – Use cucumber, tomatoes, lettuce, fennel, peppers, onions
  - ◊ Blend all the ingredients together
  - ◊ (Don't cook this one – it is jolly good raw and cold)
  - ◊ Again, check the carbs in Appendix 3 (page 115 – you will know what is right for you once you have established ketosis)
  - ◊ Eat with PK bread and PK garlic butter

Historical note regarding gazpacho: *Back to the Romans! Roman legionaries used to carry dried bread, garlic and vinegar and any other pieces of salads and vegetables that they could find, to make impromptu cold, raw soups during rest periods. The idea was taken up in Southern Spain and then there was a merging with Moorish soups. This took place in the Andalusian area of Spain during the 8th century AD. As to the name, one possible theory is that it derives from the Greek word for a collection box in church (γαζοφυλακιον) where the congregation would contribute many different shaped coins, and even bread, to the church coffers, therefore being a reference to the diversity of the contents of the soup.*

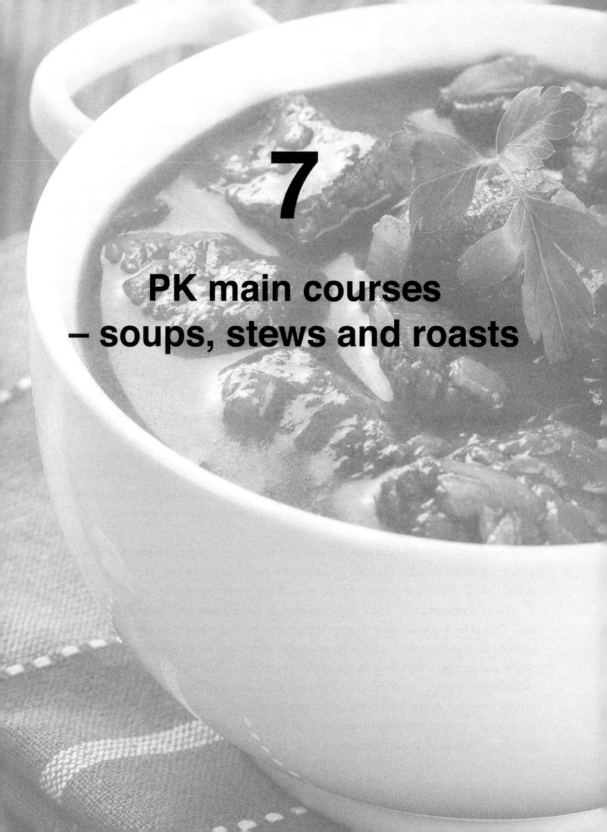

7

PK main courses
– soups, stews and roasts

Bone broth

We need brothals! *'What… we need…. is healthy fast food and the only way to provide this is to put brothals in every town, independently owned brothals that provide the basic ingredient for soups and sauces and stews. And brothals will come when … we… recognise that the food industry has prostituted itself to short cuts and huge profits, shortcuts that cheat consumers of the nutrients they should get in their food, and profits that skew the economy towards indus- trialisation in farming and food processing'* to quote the Weston A. Price Foundation.[1] In fact, I suggest a brothal in *every home*!

Linguistic and historical note: The word 'brothel' derives from the Middle English 'broth', a worthless person, and is a stem of the word 'brethen' or 'brēothan', *meaning to decay or degen- erate. Rudyard Kipling is thought to have been the originator of the phrase 'the world's oldest profession'. His 1888 story,* On the City Wall, *about a prostitute, begins with the sentence, 'Lalun is a member of the most ancient profession in the world.'*

Bone broth from boiled bones is an essential part of any PK kitchen. It formed a vital part of any mediaeval kitchen as detailed in Mrs Beeton's famous cookbook.

Mrs Beeton's Book of Household Management *(1861–65) consists of 1112 pages and con- tains over 900 recipes. Isabella Beeton (née Mayson; 14 March 1836 – 6 February 1865) said of it later: 'I must frankly own, that if I had known, beforehand, that this book would have cost me the labour which it has, I should never have been courageous enough to commence it.'*

Bone broth imparts fabulous flavour and texture to soups and stews. We acquire a taste for those things which are good for our health – see below. This makes perfect evolutionary sense and encourages us to seek out nutritious foods.

All kitchens of taste and excellence should have a stockpot permanently on the boil. This is highly efficient in terms of time and energy – bones can be added as they become available, removed after several days of boiling, by which time they will look white and parched, as if they've spent months in the Gobi desert. Don't forget you can include pigs' trotters, pigs' heads, calf's feet, oxtail, chicken bones and fish bones. Broth can be removed at any time when required for soups and stews – see below. You will be relieved to read that you do not need an open fire, a black cauldron and a witch's hat! (And although it may be fun, you do not need to recite, 'Like a hell-broth boil and bubble, Double double toil and trouble' either! (*Macbeth* Act IV, Scene 1, William Shakespeare, 26 April 1564 (baptised) – 23 April 1616).) A slow cooker does the job perfectly. I have to say that I do not even wash the stock pot out and never take it off the heat. I am lucky to have a wood-burning stove. The fact that the stove remains hot keeps it sterile so that no microbes can grow. However, if the fire goes out overnight and the stock pot cools, a solid layer of fat forms which I lift off for cooking breakfast.

Whenever I cook vegetables in water, I tip the used vegetable water into the bone broth pot to refill it as the level falls.

The benefits of bone broth
Bone broth has many directly beneficial effects, the more important of which I list below:

Bone broth for brains and immunity
Bone marrow is especially rich in micronutrients. Large mammals invested huge amounts of energy and resources to develop powerful jaws to crack open bones to access this valuable resource. We can achieve the same by boiling bones. If you wish to have good quality bone marrow (to make blood and for the immune system), together with healthy nerves, you need the raw materials for these and we can get these raw materials from bone broth.

Bone broth is a well-established treatment for recurrent infections. It is excellent for any neurological condition from autism to dementia, indeed any condition needing healing and repair, which of course is most.

Bone broth for connective tissue
Bone broth contains all the raw materials for tendons, blood vessels and coverings of internal organs. These coverings include coverings of the gut (peritoneum), the brain (meninges), the heart (pericardium), the lungs (pleural membranes), the bone (periosteum) and of course blood vessels, nerve sheaths and skin. These vital tissues have been lumped together with the boring and unimaginative title 'connective tissue'. However, connective tissue is a vital organ in its own right, seamlessly linking rock-hard bone with soft muscle and internal organs together with positively squidgy brain cells and bone marrow.

Connective tissue is vital because it holds us together but at the same time eliminates the friction between moving parts. Any such friction from physical damage or inflammation (infection, allergy, autoimmunity) results in pain and disability. Examples include peritonitis, meningitis, pericarditis, pleurisy, periostitis, costochondritis, neuritis and arteritis. Sufferers of these conditions will tell you that any movement results in severe pain because these movements are no longer without friction.

I suspect it is the mechanism of chronic friction which at least in part results in clinical pictures such as:

- bursitis: such as student's elbow, jeep bottom, housemaid's knee
- tendonitis: such as tennis elbow, golfer's elbow
- capsulitis: such as frozen shoulder
- myalgia: such as polymyalgia rheumatica.

Furthermore, the body's reaction to this friction is to prevent movement. This gives us the symptom of muscle stiffness. The starting point for treatment is bone broth.

Bone broth for leaky gut

The gut wall is held together by connective tissue. Poor quality connective tissue may result in leaky gut and all the associated problems. We seem to be seeing epidemics of hypermobility syndrome (EDS or Erlers-Danlos syndrome) often associated with chronic fatigue syndrome and, almost certainly, leaky gut. I would expect bone broth to be helpful.

Bone broth to lubricate connective tissue

Connective tissues are separated by a colloid gel which has just the right consistency to hold them together, whilst at the same time allowing them to slide without friction. These colloid gels include joint fluid (synovial fluid within the joints), cerebrospinal fluid (in the brain), pleural fluid (around the lungs) and peritoneal fluid (around the gut).

These colloid gels include substances like hyaluran and lubrican. They have an amazing property described by one of my favourite words – 'thixotropic'. The fluids become more viscous under pressure. This further protects any weight-bearing surface. Additionally, these colloid gels become less viscous with movement; this explains why muscle stiffness can be helped by movement, such as stretching or massage – this business of movement reduces the friction.

Linguistic and historical note: The word, thixotropy, derives from Ancient Greek, θιξις thixis, meaning 'touch' and τροπος, or 'tropos' meaning 'of turning'. It was invented by Herbert Freundlich originally for a sol-gel transformation. If the behaviour of fluids interests you, I am reliably informed by Craig that you should research Newtonian and non-Newtonian fluids.

Bone broth to treat arthritis and osteoporosis

Bone broth contains all the raw materials for healthy bone – a host of essential minerals such as calcium, magnesium, phosphorus, potassium, silicon, sulphur, selenium, zinc, boron, copper and manganese as well as essential building materials such as glycine, proline, arginine, various chondroitins, glucosamine, gelatin, hyaluronic acid and other such. Fish bones are rich in iodine. Gelatine is abundant in bone broth and has a long history of excellence in the treatment of arthritis and osteoporosis.

Twice-boiled chicken bones are an effective Chinese remedy for arthritis.

Bone broth for skin, hair and nails

Bone broth contains the raw materials to make keratin. This is one of the toughest proteins in Nature. Very many of my patients comment that the quality of their skin, hair and nails is greatly improved by bone broth. Indeed, nail health reflects bone health and a good DIY test for osteoporosis is to look at your nails. Hard, strong, tough-to-cut nails reflect hard, strong, difficult-to-break bones. Improved skin quality is another bonus.

Soup

Bone broth alone makes for a delicious soup. To this add PK vegetables – that is to say, low-carb vegetables or small amounts of high-carb vegetables that are in season (see Appendix 3, page 115).

I am extremely fortunate in having a vegetable garden – failing that or an allotment (and the time to do the gardening), organise a regular vegetable box delivery from a local grower. We have a fantastic local system here in Radnorshire, so there must be one near you. The Soil Association would be a good place to start looking (see Appendix 5, page 125).My favourite combinations are as follows in Table 8.

Table 8: PK soups

Bone broth plus:	Seasonal suggestions of very low carb vegetables to add (see 'Green list', Appendix 3, page 117)	Seasonal suggestions of higher carb vegetables to add (see 'Amber list', Appendix 3, page 118) – use sparingly	As much as you like of:
Leftover veg in fridge	Lots of green leafy	Small amounts only – weigh them	Salt, pepper, garlic Spices: paprika, ginger etc. Herb garnish: parsley, rosemary, thyme etc Coconut milk to enrich
Whatever is in the garden, or whatever arrives in your veg box	Spring: Not much is available – this is the 'hungry gap' but there are treats: purple sprouting, asparagus	The 'hungry gap'	Ditto
Ditto	Summer: lettuce, tomato, green beans, courgettes, spinach, calabrese	Broad beans, onions, beetroot	Ditto
Ditto	Autumn: runner beans, mushrooms (now is the time to learn about wild mushrooms. No, I am not telling you where I find mine!)	Artichokes, carrots, squash	Ditto
Ditto	Winter: cabbage, kale, green leek tops	Parsnips, potato, white leek bottoms	Ditto
Whatever I am bad at growing in the garden	Celery, celeriac, fennel, peppers	Swede, sprouts	Ditto
Whatever is in the pantry	Tinned tomatoes Tinned prawns, shrimps Salami	Tinned beans	Ditto

Stews

The formula for making good stews is the same regardless of the meat used. Again bone broth is an essential element. However, what imparts additional flavour is to roll the meat in a mix of PK flour, sunshine (PK) salt (see Chapter 13) and seasoning, and flash fry it in a frying pan. This imparts another dimension of delicious flavour. (Don't overdo the flash frying – burnt meat has a reputation for carcinogenesis. Meats cooked in the oven at low temperatures are safe. Indeed, this is how the Japanese traditionally cook meats and Japan has more centenarians than any other country in the world.)

Table 9: The formula for PK stews

Cut meat up into chunks. The cheaper the cut the better. Cheap cuts are tough because they have more connective tissue, but this adds flavour. Include any bones. I love neck of lamb or oxtail.	Roll lumps of meat into a PK spice mix…	Flash fry in …	Flash fry…	Tip meat and onions into casserole dish
Beef, pork, lamb, goat, venison. Chicken, pheasant, guinea fowl	…linseed or coconut flour, Sunshine salt and pepper. Spices: cumin, coriander, ginger Herbs : rosemary, thyme, etc	…Lard (beef, pork, lamb) Coconut oil Palm oil PK butter is good for poultry	…Onions and garlic with leftover PK spice mix	Cover with bone broth. Leave to cook all day. A large batch lasts days! Freeze excess. Yum yum!

Roasts

The joy of a roast is that it is so quick and easy. You just stick the meat in the oven. Meat for roasting is always expensive because it reflects the ease of cooking. Again roasts are all cooked to a simple formula which is as shown in Table 10:

Table 10: The formula for PK roasts

Basic steps	Tricks of the trade
Take a lump of meat – beef, pork, lamb, venison, chicken, duck, goose, pheasant	With pork dishes, cut off the skin together with a layer of fat. The skin I cook separately to make perfect crackling. If the skin is cooked on the joint you risk eating good crackling and dry meat, or perfect meat and soggy crackling! Why not have good crackling and perfect meat?
Place in roasting tray and cover with lard	The flavour is in the fat – ideally use strips of peritoneal or leaf fat. This leaves delicious crispy scratchings on the top of the joint. I generally scoff these before they get to the table.
Put a whole onion into the roasting tin	Leave the onion skin on – this imparts great flavour and browns the gravy. (Thank you Rosemary for that tip!)
Put in a hot oven, say 220°C. Set the timer for 30 minutes.	The cooks tell me this 'seals' the outside of the joint and stops flavour leaking out. I am not so sure this is correct but hey ho – it works in practice!
When the timer goes off, take the joint out of oven and baste with the fat which will have run off. Reduce the temperature to 180 degrees. Reset timer – see opposite for timings.	The total cooking time should be about 20 minutes per pound (half kilo), but less if it is a very large joint. With experience you will get a feel for this.
When the timer goes off, remove the joint from the oven and lift onto a carving dish. Cover it with grease proof paper and a towel. Allow it to 'rest' for 30 minutes.	The meat continues to cook at this very low temperature without drying out and the meat remains succulent.
Turn your attention back to the roasting tin. Pick up the onion and squeeze the soft centre out. Chuck the outside of the onion into the bone broth pot. Add garlic to the tin. Add bone broth. Put on to the cooker and heat; mash the onion in and scrape the brown bits off the bottom. Stir.	The most gorgeous gravy results. Serve. Use PK bread to mop up the juices if there are not enough veg to do the job. Or worse, I suggest my dining companions look away, tip the plate up and slurp excess gravy up direct. It makes an impolite noise, but is another highlight of my meal! The dog looks on anxiously to make sure I do not lick the plate too…

You are now well on your way to becoming a PK cook. As Craig's Nan used to say to him, when giving advice on possible brides: 'Kissing don't last; cookery do.' In fact, Nan Robinson was quoting George Meredith, English novelist and poet (12 February 1828 – 18 May 1909), from his novel *The Ordeal of Richard Feverel* (1859).

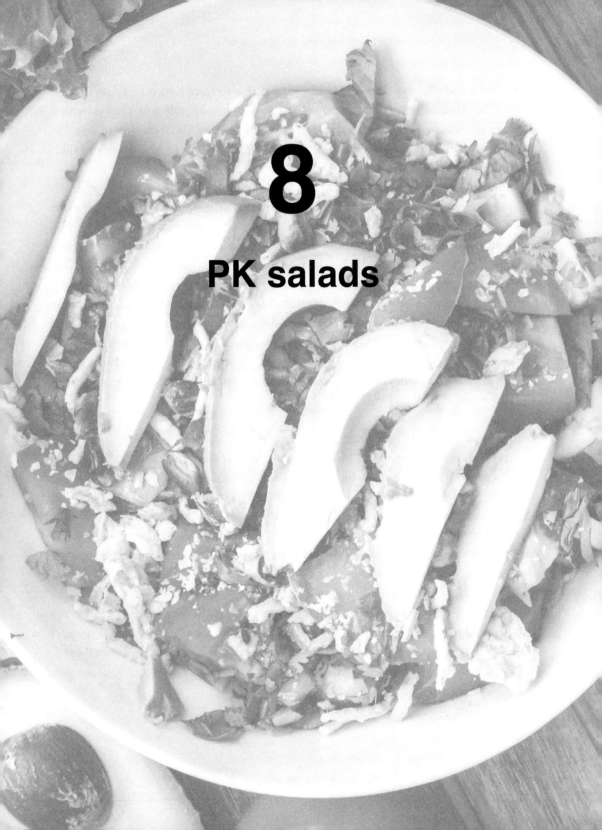

8

PK salads

The word 'salad' derives from the Latin 'sal' (salt), a form of which is 'salata' (salted things). In classical times, raw vegetables were eaten with salt and always with a dressing of vinegar or oil, and this dish was called 'salata'. The inclusion of an oil in the 'salads' of the Romans and Greeks gives us a first clue as to how modern salads should be prepared.

Another clue comes from Lucius Junius Moderatus Columella (4–70 AD), generally regarded as the most important writer on agriculture in the Roman empire, who, in his 12-volume *Res Rustica*, recommends the inclusion of eggs and nuts to 'salata'.

I routinely ask my patients about their diet. Invariably the reply, 'Well, I eat lots of salad', is accompanied by a smug smile. Oh dear… I am going to have to disillusion you. Salads may satisfy your palate and conscience but they will not satisfy your appetite. One cannot be well nourished by salad alone. Modern Western salads not only lack fuel in the form of fibre and fat, but they also lack goodness in the form of protein and micronutrients. We have salad vegetables to entertain us, not to nourish us. I will not bore you with a list of salad vegetables, but think of lettuce, cucumber, tomato, pepper,… yawn… yawn. Wake up! Don't forget raw cabbage, carrot, beetroot… cheap with the great 'crunch factor'. We call it coleslaw.

The importance of sound ('the crunch factor') in our enjoyment of eating has been confirmed in the paper 'Eating with our ears' by C Spence. Spence looked at the crispiness and crunchiness of many food types, from salads to bacons to the crackle that one senses when drinking sparkling water. He even went on to investigate the distinctive 'cracking' sound at the first bite of the Magnum ice cream – when a new formula was tried for Magnum, which reduced this cracking sound, sales fell dramatically. I am not *suggesting you should be eating Magnum ice creams, but the point remains that sounds are an important part of the taste and eating experience and salads provide this 'crunch'.*

So, the redeeming features of salad are taste and texture – variety and crunch are satisfying and enhance the eating experience. However, for salad to be a useful part of the PK diet, we must refer back to the classical era; salads need to be fortified by:

1. A good oily salad dressing (if you do not have the time or energy to make one, then buy one).
2. Added fibre, fat, protein and micronutrients.

1. Salad dressing

Always make a large batch of your chosen dressing because it keeps so well in the fridge.

Put the following into your Nutribullet, or equivalent:

Table 11: The formula for PK salad dressings

Essentials for French dressing	Large dollop of oil	In order of preference I use olive, hemp, rapeseed, safflower, or sesame oil. Usually cold-pressed 'virgins'!
	Same amount of lemon or lime juice	And/or …if you are not allergic to yeast, then add in cider or white wine vinegar
	Garlic – at least one clove. Usually three or four. (I love garlic!)	'Lazy garlic' is quicker, but not quite so good
	Level teaspoon sunflower lecithin	This emulsifies and blends the oil and water-based components
	Large pinch of 'sunshine salt' (see page 93) to provide all the essential minerals plus vitamins D and B12. Pepper	Whizz it all up together
Extras	Teaspoon of grain mustard…	…or horseradish sauce (or horseradish root from the garden) or piece of fresh ginger
	If you are well within your carb allowance (see page 115)…	…then a ½ teaspoon of treacle as this imparts great texture
To make mayonnaise	Add in two egg yolks	Whizz it all up together
To make hollandaise	Instead of egg yolks, add a dollop of Grace coconut milk	Whizz it all up together

Use this dressing liberally on all your salads.

2. Salad dressing with added extras for fibre, fat, protein and micronutrients

Table 12: The formula for sustaining PK salads

Fat	To add to any of the alternative dressings in Table 11: Avocado Pork scratchings (these are surprisingly good in salad)
Fibre	PK vegetables (see Appendix 3, page 115) PK nuts: walnuts, brazils, pecans, almonds (see Appendix 3, page 115). PK seeds: sunflower, pumpkin, sesame (see Appendix 3, page 115, for the carb content)
Protein	Boiled eggs Quorn, tofu Corned beef, chunks of salami, cold meat, biltong Smoked fish, fish such as tuna, sardines, mackerel, salmon (tinned, fresh or frozen – I usually use tinned) Prawns, shrimps, anchovies, cockles, mussels (tinned, fresh or frozen)
Minerals, vitamins D and B12	Sunshine salt – a generous pinch

The Golden Rule: Keep it quick, simple and easy. I am idle and I expect the rest of you to be so too – or just exhausted. If you are challenged by energy, time or inclination, buy prepared salad, pour on hemp oil and generously sprinkle with sunshine salt.

Point of historical interest: Virgil (70-19 BC) wrote briefly about the preparation of salads in his work Moretum. *He says:*

> *It manus in gyrum; paullatim singula vires*
> *Deperdunt proprias; color est E pluribus unus.*

Which translates as:
  Spins round the stirring hand; lose by degrees
  Their separate powers the parts, and comes at last,
  From many several colours, one that rules.

So, the motto of the United States of America, *E pluribus unum*, is in fact an instruction in a salad recipe!

9

Lard, dripping and fat

'Fat is the most valuable food known to man.'
John Yudkin (8 August 1910 – 12 July 1995), Professor of Nutrition and Diabetes,
Queen Elizabeth College, London University, UK

John Yudkin's book, Pure, White and Deadly *(1972), summarised the dangers of sugar consumption – namely, an increased incidence of coronary thrombosis, obesity, diabetes, liver disease, and some cancers. It is well worth a read; his work has stood the test of time, but disastrously for the health of the Western World, Professor Yudkin's opinion was discarded in favour of that of an American nutritionist called Ancel Keys. Keys was backed by the World Sugar Research Organisation, the British Sugar Bureau and, surprise, surprise, Coca Cola. Guess who won?*

Lard, dripping and meat fat have become the cause of phobias thanks to the brainwashing propaganda of the food, margarine and Big Pharma industries. Big Pharma has implanted in the collective brain a mantra that saturated fats cause high cholesterol and high cholesterol damages arteries. The fact that there is no good evidence to support this nonsense seems to matter little when big business, money and profits get in the way. Do read our book *Prevent & Cure Diabetes*, which delivers an intellectual broadside to blow away and sink these big, fat, cholesterol lies. Perhaps Mr Sprat explains part of the reason for his physical weakness…

Jack Sprat could eat no fat,
His wife could eat no lean;
And so between them both, you see
They licked the platter clean.

English nursery rhyme

Historical note: *An early version of this rhyme appeared in John Clarke's collection of sayings in 1639. Jack Sprat was an expression for people of small stature in 16th-century England.*

Lard and meat fat are inexpensive saturated fats but they do vary greatly as regards quality – for good lard you need to shop wisely. The quality of the lard is determined by the life of the animal. Lard from free-range, grass-fed, organic, mature animals will be far superior to that from intensively reared animals. It is worth putting much effort into establishing a great source of lard. I am fortunate in having free-range pigs who can supply me.

Note from Craig: I have never seen (actually heard – see next sentence) such happy pigs as those residing at Upper Weston. They are constantly oinking – scientists from the universities of Lincoln and Belfast studied 72 male and female juvenile pigs and concluded that happier pigs and those with more curious temperaments grunt and squeal more than their less happy, less curious cousins.[1]

What was the animal fed?

'You are what you eat' applies to animals as well as *Homo sapiens*.

Origin of this phrase: There are many possibilities but the earliest modern verified reference is that of Anthelme Brillat-Savarin who wrote, in Physiologie du Gout, ou Meditations de Gastronomie Transcendante, *1826: 'Dis-moi ce que tu manges, je te dirai ce que tu es.' [Tell me what you eat and I will tell you what you are.] (Anthelme Brillat-Savarin, 1 April 1755 – 2 February 1826, was a French lawyer and politician, and later an epicure and gastronome.)*

So you need to know what the animal was fed. Pigs fed on fish meal taste of fish! These pigs have to be swapped to a grain-based diet for at least two weeks before slaughter. Where I live here in Radnorshire, all sheep and beef stock live free range on the hills. Their fat is always delicious.

Buy leaf (peritoneal,* gut) or kidney fat

Professor Caroline Pond, in her book *The Fats of Life*, details how fat is laid down where the immune system is busy. This makes perfect evolutionary sense – the immune system is greatly demanding of energy and raw materials such as zinc, selenium and iodine. All these commodities need to be readily available for when the immune system is challenged. Furthermore, taste evolved for very good reasons – it allows us to select the most nutritious foods (be careful not to confuse *taste* with *addiction* that drive us to eat the wrong things!). So, it is no coincidence that 90 per cent of the immune system is associated with the gut (because the gut is heaving with microbes), and peritoneal, gut or 'leaf' fat has the best flavour. Indeed, when I go to the butchers I

*Footnote: The peritoneum is a layer of thin tissue that lines the abdomen and covers all of the organs within it, such as the bowel and the liver.

ask for the lumpy leaf fat. Because it is not attractive, either physically or socially, I am often asked if I want it to feed the birds. 'Oh yes,' say I, thinking that the old buzzard standing in front of the gorgeous young butcher is to be the main recipient.

Indeed, following visits to the butcher you can look forward to three cheap and delicious products: good lard, scratchings and rillette.

Buy rendered fat

You can purchase excellent lards and dripping online, such as free-range Berkshire pork fat, beef fat, duck fat and goose fat. However, if you do have the time and energy to render your own, then you are in for the discovery of a lifetime – proper scratchings!

Render you own fat *and* make scratchings

If any food should be a 'super food', this is it. When you purchase large chunks of leaf fat, you are not just buying lard. You are also buying peritoneal membranes which hold it all together alongside lymph nodes and lymphatics. These latter items are highly nutritious and make for the most divine scratchings.

Making dripping is a job that can be done in large batches since it will keep for weeks in the fridge and months in the deep freeze.

- Cut the leaf fat into strips no thicker that one centimetre.
- Spread them out on a wire rack over an oven tray and place in the oven at 180°C.
- As the fat melts onto the oven tray, pour it off into a pot. Keep doing this until no more fat runs. It should produce white fat – if the fat is brown then the oven is too hot.
- Allow to cool and store in the fridge and/or freezer.

You will be left with brown 'scratchings' on the wire rack, which you should lift off. Serve these with sunshine salt (see page 98). In my family, major wars would erupt if the distribution of scratchings was not seen to be entirely fair. We would all oversee the division of them into four equal piles. We would then pick straws for who took which pile. The next stage of proceedings was to savour each mouthful and see who could eat them the slowest – and then tease the eater-uppers with that final delicious mouthful. One ploy would be to secrete a morsel without the others noticing… then triumphantly reveal this when all else had been consumed. Indeed, we used this method to split up the contents of our Mum's house, after she died, into four heaps. It resulted in a hilarious afternoon from what could have been a sombre and miserable job – I am sure she would have approved!

In Craig's house things are much more sedate, due to there being two resident mathematicians. For dividing into two equal piles, for example, the procedure is that one person divides the food into two piles and the other person chooses which pile they want. This encourages the 'divider' to divide equally. More complicated methods, from set theory, apply for dividing into three and four piles. Amazingly, Craig and Gina normally end up with bigger piles than Penny and Conor, but it is all done completely fairly according to set theory... those who are interested may like to read 'Fair cake-cutting' on Wikipedia, although cakes are most definitely not 'PK'!

Commercial poor scratchings are made as above but the pork skin is included. This can make them tough.

Rillette

I make rillettes (similar to paté) from my pig heads and trotters; it is important to include the eyes because anything made from such will see you through the week... boom boom! (Craig)
- Boil up the heads and trotters and allow to cool.
- Use your hands to pull off the meat, lard, fat, brains, tongue and connective tissue.
- Put this, slightly warm, into the Nutribullet and whizz up into a gloop.
- Season with sunshine salt and pepper.
- Put into the pot, then into the fridge – it will set to a firm consistency.
- Remaining bones go back into the stock pot.

You will be left with hands covered with fat. Rub this into your skin – lard is the perfect fat for skin. The sheep shearers know this too – after a day's shearing the callused hands and arms of these tough farmers become as soft as the proverbial baby's bottom. This derives from the lard that waterproofs the sheep's wool, called lanolin. (So called 'wool fat soap' was a very common traditional soap, made from lanolin. Modern versions of wool fat soap contain many additives for colour and 'fragrance' and are poor cousins to the original.)

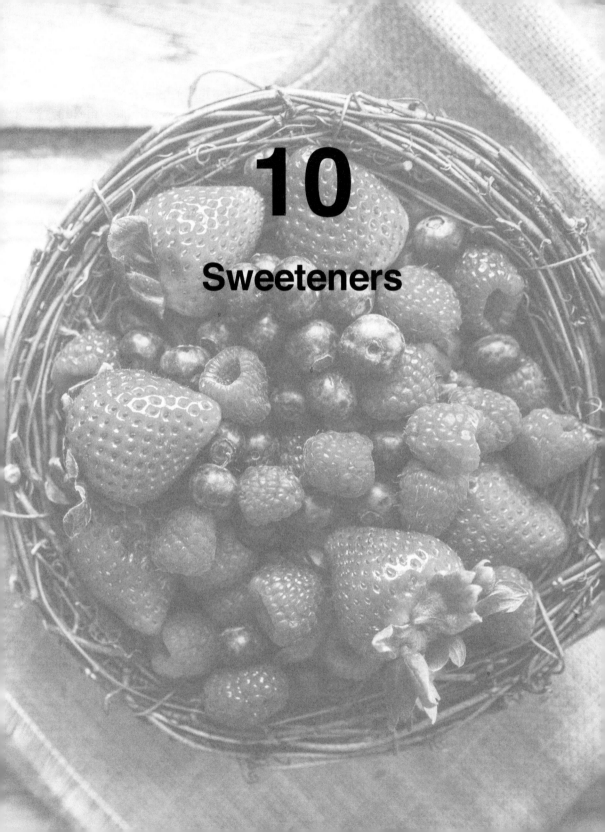

10
Sweeteners

Did I catch you out? If you find yourself turning straight to this chapter, then you have failed the keto test – you are still a sugar and carb addict. I have been through the full evolution of using various sweeteners and have come to the conclusion that none can be permitted.

'thy sweet deceiving, Lock me in delight awhile.'

John Fletcher, playwright, 1579 – 1625

This is how it is with sweeteners; they 'deceive' us through a variety of means, which we often perceive as a 'delight', and here the addiction begins and continues. So, no sweeteners are allowed for the following reasons:

1. 'Old habits die hard' (Old English Proverb)

Sweeteners, whether real or artificial, prevent the palate from changing away from craving sweetness. But, change it can, will and does. One such example is the sugar addict who has successfully, and for some time, stopped sweetening his tea – now any sugar taste in his tea seems disgustingly sweet. I find I can now eat blackcurrants (admittedly with coconut milk) without my mouth puckering up with the sharpness – for me this is a real change.

In a sense, for some, this whole book will be about stopping old (bad) habits and starting new (good) ones. So, we pause for a moment and take a step back. There are many books available on how to embed 'good habits' into your psyche. I won't recommend one over the other as we are all different. But there are some common threads:

- It can be difficult but is always very worthwhile.
- The behavioural scientists give this changeover from 'old' to 'new' habits a name, 'habit formation', and generally it is agreed that habit formation can take some considerable time for some people. Lally et al reported in 2010 that the average time for participants to reach the point where the 'new' habit becomes 'automatic' is 66 days, with a range of 18–254 days. This point of 'automaticity' is where the 'new' habit does not have to be reinforced or even thought about – it happens 'naturally'.
- I do like the well-known three-word encapsulation of the process of habit formation, 'Reminder, Repeat, Reward' – the three Rs. In this context, the 'reminder' is when we go to eat, the 'repeat' is when we follow the guidelines

in this book [!] and the 'reward' is the healthier person we become.

• But, really I can't put it better than Aristotle [Note from Craig – who can?!]

'We are what we repeatedly do. Excellence, then, is not an act, but a habit.'

Aristotle, 384 BC – 322 BC

[Sarah – Aristotle is only right so long as the habit is the right one… Craig – sigh… .]

2. The Pavlovian response

The body is intelligent. It knows that a sugar hit will require an insulin spike to deal with it. It has learned this from experience, and so anticipates the sugar spike from a sweet taste in the mouth and pours out insulin in response to such. Artificial sweeteners will therefore spike insulin and switch off fat burning and so push you back into the metabolic hinterland, where there is no fuel available from carbs and you cannot burn fat because insulin is high. This explains why artificial sweeteners are so counter-productive in calorie restricted diets.

Historical note: Ivan Pavlov (26 September 1849 – 27 February 1936) played the sound of a metronome to dogs and afterwards gave them food. After a few repetitions the dogs associated the noise of the metronome with food and so would salivate merely on the sound of the metronome even in the absence of food. This is much like rustling a packet of crisps at Craig – he will salivate! Pavlov went on to report more observations about this 'Pavlovian response'; for example, the 'conditioning' happened more quickly when the interval between the sound of the metronome and the food was shortest during the initial period when the dogs were being 'conditioned'.

3. It's all or nothing!

Note: It seems like there is a day for everything now. Apparently 26 July is 'It's All or Nothing Day' (www.nationaldaycalendar.com) (Craig: I think there should be a day reserved as 'This day is not a special day for anything' Day… but that would make it special too…)

A sweet taste hit switches on a sugar craving in the same way that the whiff of tobacco smoke may switch on the desire for a fag in nicotine addicts. We all know that smokers have to stop smoking completely – they cannot be satisfied with one puff a day. The same is true of alcoholics – they celebrate complete abstinence because they know this is the only way to cure their addiction. They have no 'off' button so do not dare switch it 'on' in the first place.

4. 'A sweet poison' (old English saying)

'The "sweet poison of the false infinite"'

CS Lewis, 29 November 1898–22 November 1963

Artificial sweeteners are toxic in their own right. Aspartame is metabolised in the liver to formaldehyde, which is a neurotoxin and indeed a pesticide. I remain convinced that a 39-year-old woman who consulted me had her motor neurone disease triggered by a diet which saw her replace all sweeteners with aspartame – we reckoned she had consumed over a kilogram of the stuff during a few months. This was the youngest case of MND I had (and have) ever seen.

The studies are beginning to come through showing the dangers of aspartame – see for example Rycerz & Jaworska-Adamu, 2013.[2] They concluded that: 'Despite intense speculations about the carcinogenicity of aspartame, the latest studies show that its metabolite – diketopiperazine – is carcinogenic in the CNS [central nervous system]. It contributes to the formation of tumours in the CNS such as gliomas, medulloblastomas and meningiomas.'

Moreover, in the paper by Soffritti et al (2014) of the Cesare Maltoni Cancer Research Center, Ramazzini Institute, Bologna, Italy, the authors concluded that: 'On the basis of the evidence of the potential carcinogenic effects of APM (aspartame) herein reported, a re-evaluation of the current position of international regulatory agencies must be considered an urgent matter of public health.'[3]

5. Sugar alcohols

'I pray you, do not fall in love with me, For I am falser than vows made in wine.'
As You Like It, Rosalind in Act 3 Scene V, William Shakespeare, 26 April 1564 (baptised) – 23 April 1616

Sugar alcohols, such as xylitol, run into the same problems as described above. Whilst they may not increase blood sugar levels, I would expect them to increase blood sugar alcohol levels. My guess is that these are as toxic as sugar in the bloodstream.

Note: Sugar alcohols are neither sugars nor alcohol – isn't organic chemistry wonderful? For those who are interested, here are some definitions:

- *Sugar alcohols – These are organic compounds, that are typically derived from sugars. A sugar alcohol is neither a sugar nor an alcohol – see below. They are white, water-soluble solids that can occur naturally or are often produced industrially from sugars. They are used widely in the food industry as thickeners and sweeteners.*
- *Blood sugar level – Sometimes known as the blood sugar concentration or blood glucose level, this is the amount of glucose (sugar) present in the blood of a human or animal. It is generally measured in millimoles per litre.*
- *Blood sugar alcohol level – This is the amount of sugar alcohol present in the blood of a human or animal.*

There is some evidence that sugar alcohols do affect blood sugar levels although less so than sugars (see references 4 and 5).

Finally, here are the structures of sugars, alcohols and sugar alcohols for those who remember their school chemistry:

- *Sugars – These can take many forms. 'Monosaccharides' have the general formula $C_6H_{12}O_6$ – that is, five hydroxyl groups (–OH) and a carbonyl group (C=O). 'Disaccharides' have the general formula $C_{12}H_{22}O_{11}$. They are formed by the combination of two monosaccharide molecules.*
- *Alcohols – These again can take many forms and can be primary or secondary alcohols. The simplest primary alcohol is methanol (CH_3OH). Essentially an alcohol is an organic compound in which the hydroxyl functional group (–OH) is bound to a saturated carbon atom. A carbon atom is called saturated if there are only single 'bonds' between it and other atoms – that is, there are no carbon-carbon double bonds or triple bonds.*
- *Sugar alcohols – Sugar alcohols have the general formula $HOCH_2(CHOH)_nCH_2OH$ whereas sugars have two fewer hydrogen atoms – for example, $HOCH_2(CHOH)_nCHO$ or $HOCH_2(CHOH)_{n-1}C(O)CH_2OH$.*

Now for those at the back of the class, stop passing silly notes and wake up!

Summary

When people tell me they do not like a particular food, I ask them to analyse what they mean by 'like'. The answer should relate to taste, texture (crunch or chew factors) and/or smell (something familiar or evocative). However, many people 'like' a food because it provides a psychological hit. They are often unaware of this mechanism and refuse to admit to it. Without a sugar or carb rush, the meal does not satisfy. Take the sugar rush out and junk food reverts to the bland, tasteless, nutritionally criminal mush that it is.

You can give up your addiction to sweeteners; what I have explained gives the intellectual imperative to do so. Then you must dig deep and find the will within yourself to 'kick the habit'. Once kicked, you will wonder why you were ever 'hooked'. But remember, the time to do this is now!

'Carpe diem' – *'Seize the day'*

Book 1, Odes, Horace, 65 BC – 8 BC

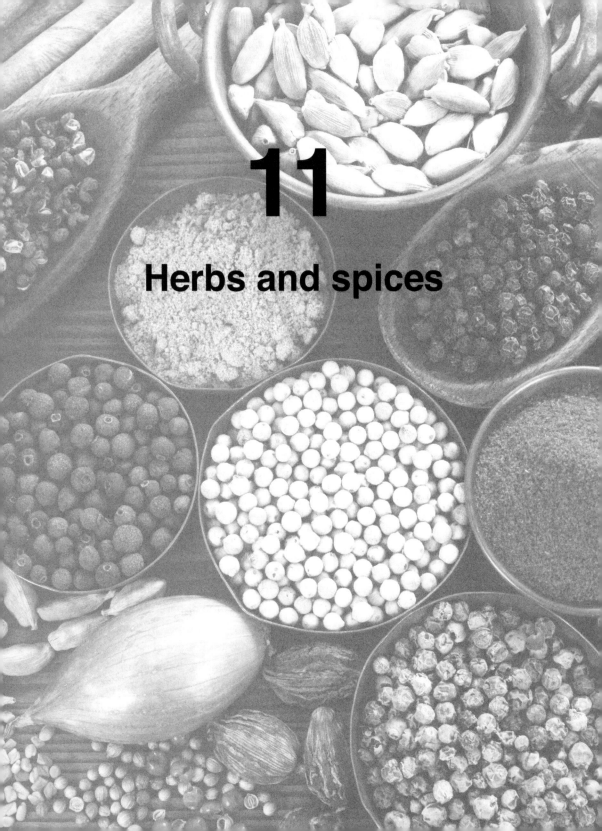

11

Herbs and spices

Of US policy in the early stages of the Cold War, regarding 'winning' the nuclear arms race, Churchill said:

> 'If you go on with this nuclear arms race, all you are going to do is make the rubble bounce.'

Sir Winston Leonard Spencer-Churchill, KG OM CH TD PC DL FRS RA,
30 November 1874 – 24 January 1965

Churchill was making the point that such an arms race was not 'winnable', as such.

It is similar for the arms race going on inside our bodies – we can never totally eradicate the bad guys and 'win', but we can keep ahead of the game. This arms race is a 'numbers game' – our body must use its 'resources' to keep the numbers of the bad guys (that is, harmful microbes) down to a sufficiently low level so that we stay well. We must do what we can to help our bodies. That this constant battle is going on is clear – within minutes of death, when our bodies cease fighting this arms race, we rapidly decompose; the bad guys win, and they win quickly. (For much more on this, please see my book, *Sustainable Medicine – Whistle blowing on 21st century medical practice* and also my webpage.)

So, life itself is an arms race. You and I represent a potential free lunch for the myriad of bacteria, moulds, parasites, worms, yeasts and viruses which are constantly straining to make themselves at home in our warm, comfortable bodies. Throughout Evolution, infections have been major killers. We imagine we have won that arms race with modern hygiene, antimicrobials, drugs and vaccinations. Wrong! We have been lulled into a false sense of security by drug company propaganda. We know that low-grade chronic infections are driving many chronic pathologies, such as autoimmunity (one in every 20 Westerners has an autoimmune condition), allergy, arthritis and chronic fatigue syndrome (CFS). Indeed, many of our major killers may have their roots in infection. More recently it has become apparent that many cases of CFS/ME (myalgic encephalitis) are driven by new infections – microbes that have made themselves at home because the defences of our bodies are generally declining. These microbes include Lyme disease (borrelia), bartonella, babesia, mycoplasmas, chlamydia, erlicha, yersinia and rickettsia, and possibly others. The herpes viruses in particular target the brain and the immune system, and increasingly I am finding many CFS/ME patients improve with antimicrobials against bacteria, viruses, yeasts, parasites and, in some cases, worms. Yeast infections are becoming pandemic so it now seems almost routine that babies have oral thrush. (Please see the chapter on Lyme disease and other co-infections in our books *Diagnosis and Treatment of Chronic Fatigue Syndrome and Myalgic Encephalitis* and *The Natural Treatment of Infection*.)

Common causes of death and related infections

Table 13: Common causes of death and their infectious associates

Disease		Associated microbes	Notes
Cancer	Breast, womb, ovary	HHV 3 (chicken pox and shingles)	The Pill and HRT constitute the largest risk for these cancers and many others
	Mouth	HHV 1 (*Herpes simplex* – cold sores)	Alcohol is also a major risk
	Oesophageal	Microbes in the upper fermenting gut. These are a major cause of acid reflux. HPV-16 (human papilloma virus)	We are seeing epidemics of Barratt's oesophagus – a premalignant condition. I now have 3 patients whose Barratt's has resolved on a PK diet
	Stomach	*Helicobacter-pylori* HHV4 (Epstein Barr virus – glandular fever)	*H pylori* can be abolished with antibiotics—herbal treatments may also be effective. This microbe is usually picked up during childhood.
	Colon	Abnormal microbiome Associated with inflammatory bowel disease (IBD)	IBS can be caused by an abnormal gut microbiome. The PK diet is highly effective at treating IBS
	Cervical	HHV 2 (genital herpes) HPV (human papilloma virus – genital warts)	The Pill and HRT constitute the largest risk for this cancer. Not only are they growth promoting but also immuno-suppressive.
	Prostate	HHV 5 (cytomegalovirus)	Dairy products contain growth promotors – see chapter 4 on PK dairy. This may explain the low incidence of prostate cancer in China.

Disease		Associated microbes	Notes
	Lymphoma and leukaemia	HTLV 1 (human T lymphotropic virus) HHV 4 (Epstein Barr virus – glandular fever) HHV 6	Gut lymphoma is associated with coeliac disease – further reason to avoid gluten grains!
	Brain	HHV 5 (cytomegalovirus). There is a 90% association with glioblastoma. HHV 6	The PK diet is the starting point to treat all brain pathologies! There are cases in the medical literature of malignant glioblastomas being effectively treated with PK diets.[1]
	Liver	Hepatitis B Hepatitis C	
Alzheimer's disease, Parkinson's		HHV 1 (*Herpes simplex* – cold sores) HHV 4 (Epstein Barr virus – glandular fever) HHV 6 Lyme disease (borreliosis)	There is a clear link with herpes,[2] but… …the greatest cause is metabolic syndrome (loss of control of blood sugar due to cells becoming insensitive to insulin – the precursor to type-2 diabetes) – indeed, Alzheimer's has been dubbed 'type-3 diabetes'(see our book *Prevent and Cure Diabetes*)
Arterio-sclerosis	Major cause of heart disease and strokes[3]	Chlamydia pneumoniae HHV 5 (cytomegalovirus)	The greatest cause is metabolic syndrome – again, see our book *Prevent and Cure Diabetes*
Multiple sclerosis		HHV 4 (Epstein Barr virus – glandular fever) HHV 6	There are many other environmental factors involved, especially toxic metals like mercury

Please see the website of the American Cancer Society for more detail.[4]

Protecting ourselves against infection

The PK diet is highly protective against all infection. The vast majority of infections get into our bodies through the mouth (food and water) and nose (inhalation). Inhaled microbes stick to the mucous lining of the nose and bronchi and this mucus is coughed up and swallowed. All these microbes should end up in the acid bath of the stomach where they are killed. This acid bath works best when the stomach is empty because the acid is concentrated. Dilute this acid bath with food and you provide a susceptible window of opportunity for these microbes to invade. If that food is high in carbohydrate then you additionally feed these microbes. That leaves us with a susceptible window when we eat food. This is one reason snacking is so bad for us, especially high-carb snacking, and why having two meals a day is so advantageous. This makes the PK diet highly protective against all infection. We can, however, improve matters even more with herbs and spices.

Craig recommends the play The Herbal Bed, *a period piece about Shakespeare's daughter, who is accused of adultery. I won't give any more away but crucial to the plot is the emphasis on the healing properties of herbs both to specific ailments and also to general health. These properties have been known for centuries and are well expounded in this brilliantly written play. We toss aside our ancestors' wisdom at our peril.*

If you look at life from the point of view of a plant, it does not want to be eaten. Plants cannot run away like prey animals – their only defence is to make themselves as unpalatable as possible. All plants are stuffed with natural antimicrobials: antihelminthics (helminths are types of worm), antiparasitics, antibacterials, antifungals and antivirals. Indeed, if any plant were lacking any such defences, it would have been overcome by such at some point in evolution. Plants are all survivors. The key to good health and cooking is to choose those which poison the invaders instead of us – and taste great! Indeed, many gorgeous Indian spices were used primarily to preserve food between harvesting and eating when it would otherwise go off in a hot climate.

'Let food be thy medicine and medicine be thy food'

Hippocrates, 'father of medicine', 460–370 BC

I see many patients with chronic fatigue syndrome and it is increasingly becoming apparent that chronic infection is a major player. Some do very well with anti-invader drugs. However, I am impressed by how well the herbal regimes work. Both regimes are most effective when combined with a PK diet. Sometimes we have to do it all – drugs, herbals and diet to get a result.

'Bernard was right; the pathogen is nothing; the terrain is everything.'

Louis Pasteur (1822 – 1895) – deathbed words

With the PK diet and judicious use of herbs and spices, we are changing the terrain in our favour.

Historical note: Pasteur had five children with his wife, Marie Laurent. Only two of their children survived to adulthood; the other three died of typhoid. These personal tragedies were a major motivation for Pasteur's work. Like many geniuses, Pasteur was fearless. Just as Sir Isaac Newton risked his eyesight by staring at the sun – I do not advise this of course! – in order to confirm his theories as laid out in The Optiks, *so did Pasteur take risks for his voyage of scientific discovery. In* The Story of San Michele, *Munthe writes: 'Pasteur himself was absolutely fearless. Anxious to secure a sample of saliva straight from the jaws of a rabid dog, I once saw him with the glass tube held between his lips draw a few drops of the deadly saliva from the mouth of a rabid bull-dog, held on the table by two assistants, their hands protected by leather gloves.'*

Which herbs and spices to use?

I do not think this matters much so long as you use them. All plants show anti-invader activity and indeed the herbal textbooks list a multiplicity of actions for every spice and herb. Sometimes it is difficult to know where to start. It's a bit like exercise – unless you like doing it you will conveniently forget, so use the ones you like and use lots of them. People who complain that the PK diet is boring will be less able to do so once armed with herbs and spices. Everyone will have their own personal list but our favourites are as follows:

Table 14: Recommendations for using herbs and spices

Food	What to add	Comments
Meat	Pepper – a lot of it	Pepper is a rich source of zinc – zinc deficiency is extremely common! During the 16th century pepper was a currency preferred more than gold.
	Sunshine salt	This supplies all essential minerals for the immune system to fight invaders. See chapter 13
	Garlic – a lot of it	Garlic supplements are the most consumed supplement in Germany due to garlic's multiple health benefits – it is especially protective against heart and arterial disease

PK butter (see page 33)	Garlic	To make garlic bread – yum yum
PK French dressing (see page 59)	Garlic Olive oil Sunshine salt	
Lamb	Cook with a large handful of rosemary	Antibacterial and antioxidant. A long-living community on a Greek island – Ikaria - who have no Alzheimer's, attribute their longevity to living on a hillside (exercise) and rosemary.[5]
Pork	Cook up cranberries – gently boil until rendered down into thick sauce	The sharpness of these sauces is an exquisite contrast and balance to the fat of pork
Beef	Horseradish sauce and wasabi	Good anti-cancer properties
Curry dishes	Ginger	A medicinal spice widely used in Chinese medicine
	Cardamom, cumin, coriander	Buy the best you can get, keep them whole and grind at the last minute. Roll the raw lump of meat in the spices and flash fry them – this releases the best flavours
PK bread	Add a teaspoon of caraway seed	
All vegetable dishes	Pour on cold-pressed olive oil – lots of it	
Onions and leeks	Turmeric powder sprinkled on – lots of it	Curcumin is the active ingredient of turmeric and widely used in many gut conditions as an anti-inflammatory.[6]
Cabbage	Cook with caraway seeds	Good treatment for the fermenting gut
Tomato	Basil	
Crumble toppings	Cinnamon – lots of it Nutmeg	Anti-inflammatory, improves brain function, anti-cancer
Tea …	Black tea, green tea. Ginger tea [others]	These are the only substances you should consume between your two main meals. Most have antimicrobial activity and help keep the upper gut 'clean and tidy'.

...and coffee	...but do not over-do!	Improves brain function in the short term

Herbs to counter established infections

If I have a patient with an established infection, such as Lyme disease, chlamydia or chronic fungal infection, then there are three herbs that I routinely recommend. Whilst they do have direct antimicrobial actions, just as importantly they improve our defences – that is to say, they help the immune system deal with all infection regardless of the infective organism. Also, they are all very safe and can be included in our everyday PK diet because they are low carb and delicious! They are:

- Rhodiola tea – one teaspoonful with boiling water poured over it.
- Astragalus dried root – This can be eaten off the spoon and chewed until all the flavour has gone; then spit out the woody remains. It makes a reasonable chewing gum substitute. It is also delicious in stews – you can add in tablespoon amounts.
- Cordyceps sinensis – this is a fungus that grows parasitically on a particular type of caterpillar and has been used for centuries in Chinese medicine. It makes the most delicious chocolate, used with equal amounts of cocoa butter, coconut oil and cordyceps powder, imparting a flavour like chocolate with a hint of coffee and truffle. It really is quite superb – one of the best medicines ever!

Cordyceps chocolate

Ingredients
- 200 grams cocoa butter
- 200 grams coconut oil
- 200 grams cordyceps powder
- 200 grams dried goji berries

Melt the cocoa butter and coconut oil in a pan and stir in the cordyceps powder

Tip the dried goji berries into a flat plastic container (my daughter uses lots of paper cake cups) and cover them with the mix

Put in the fridge to set

Eat directly from cold.

For further evidence of the healing and disease-preventing nature of herbs and spices, the interested reader can search the online database. Sadly, not enough research has been done in this area, presumably because there are no patents and large profits to be made. However, Christine M Kaefer and John A Milner have published significantly on this.[7, 8] In Kaefer & Milner (2008), they state: 'A growing body of epidemiological and preclinical evidence points to culinary herbs and spices as minor dietary constituents with multiple anticancer characteristics,' and in their chapter in the book *Herbal Medicine: Biomolecular and Clinical Aspects*, they conclude: 'Mounting evidence suggests that cancers are not an inevitable consequence of aging but are preventable diseases. The evidence in this chapter suggests that spices may be factors in one's diet that may lower cancer risk and affect tumor behavior.' They add: 'Without question, evidence exists that multiple processes, including proliferation, apoptosis, angiogenesis, and immunocompetence, can be influenced by one or more spices.'[8] Indeed, this book (*Herbal Medicine: Biomolecular and Clinical Aspects*), published in 2011 and available online in full (see references), is a great place to start for those who wish to take this further than is needed for the purposes of this book.

12
Fermented foods

There is good evidence that people who regularly consume fermented foods live longer than those who do not.

'…and let me adde, that he that thoroughly understands the nature of Ferments and Fermentations, shall probably be much better able than he that Ignores them, to give a fair account of divers Phænomena of severall diseases (as well Feavers and others) which will perhaps be never thoroughly understood, without an insight into the doctrine of Fermentation.'

Robert Boyle FRS, 25 January 1627 – 31 December 1691

A comprehensive study by Stephanie N. Chilton et al (2015)[1] concluded that:

'Fermented foods have been a well-established part of the human diet for thousands of years, without much of an appreciation for, or an understanding of, their underlying microbial functionality, until recently. The use of many organisms derived from these foods, and their applications in probiotics, have further illustrated their impact on gastrointestinal wellbeing and diseases affecting other sites in the body. However, despite the many benefits of fermented foods, their recommended consumption has not been widely translated to global inclusion in food guides. Here, we present the case for such inclusion, and challenge health authorities around the world to consider advocating for the many benefits of these foods.'

We are told that these fermented, or 'probiotic', foods allow the gut to recolonise with friendly microbes, but there is little evidence that this is the case. The gut flora (or microbiome, as we must now call it) is remarkably stable. So this begs the question as to the mechanisms by which fermented foods are so good for longevity. There are many possibilities:

- When foods are fermented, the sugars and starches are fermented out, so fermented foods are necessarily low in, or devoid of, carbohydrates. You can pretty much eat fermented foods *ad lib* on the PK diet.
- When foods are fermented, lactic acid is produced – some sauerkrauts have a pH as low as 3.0, which means they are highly acidic. This helps to maintain the acidity of the stomach, so protecting against infection and improving digestion of protein and absorption of minerals. Sauerkraut is a great start to a meal because subsequent foods drop into the acid bath, which kills microbes that

may be present. (There will be lots in the Upper Weston kitchen!)

- Lactic acid is a good food source.
- Sauerkraut is rich in vitamin K2, which is essential for protection against osteoporosis and for the health of arteries and other blood vessels. (It directs calcium into bones and away from blood vessels, working cooperatively with vitamin D so we need to have enough of both for strong bones.)
- Fermented foods help prevent constipation, so potentially toxic foods spend less time in the gut where they can act as carcinogens.
- Fermentation is a great way of storing foods safely. If a food is teeming with friendly microbes, then the 'unfriendlies' cannot get in – this is protective against food poisoning. Indeed, my favourite ferment, namely kefir, we acquired from the Arabs (Turkic *köpür* meaning foam) who traditionally carry their milk in a leather pouch which dangles from their saddles and is permanently inoculated with kefir. Goats are milked directly into the pouch and the milk is rapidly fermented in the hot desert environment. It means these fellows do not need to carry a fridge on their camels in order to store and drink milk safely!

Note from Craig: More about pouches and ancient nomadic wisdom – BBC Radio 4 is the source of most of my useless information and the more useless it is, the more inclined it seems that my mind is to remember it. So here is another Radio 4-ism: Ancient Nomads used to place copper coins in their water pouches to keep the water free from bugs. In fact, the oldest recorded medical use of copper in this way is in the Smith Papyrus, one of the oldest books known. This Egyptian medical text, written between 2600 and 2200 BC, describes the application of copper to sterilise chest wounds and drinking water. This wisdom has been rediscovered recently in the paper by Gregor Grass et al (2011), 'Metallic copper as an antimicrobial surface'[2] and also in 'Copper kills antibiotic-resistant "nightmare" bacteria'.[3] It is also thought that small electric currents generated by the motion of the coins in the pouch may have helped with this water purification process.

- Although dairy products are not permitted on the PK diet, my guess is that the business of fermentation renders milk less toxic. At least the dangerous milk sugar lactose is fermented out, but the allergenic, growth-promoting proteins remain.

- Microbes in fermented foods should be rapidly killed, or at least rendered inert, by stomach acid. However, these dead or inert microbes may play an important part in training and programming the immune system in the gut. (Ninety per cent of the immune system is associated with the gut.) The immune system is our standing army – what better way to train an army than by offering up some opposition that cannot fight back? For more on this, please see our book *Diagnosis and Treatment of Chronic Fatigue Syndrome and Myalgic Encephalitis* and the entry on my website 'Reprogramming the immune system – where conventional and complementary medicine can come together'.
- Eating fermented foods means consuming friendly microbes in their billions, possibly hundreds of billions. This tsunami of friendly microbes physically displaces the 'unfriendlies' from the gut. We know probiotics are protective against gastroenteritis – English cricketers find them effective against 'Delhi Belly' while on tour. Since many infections get into our comfortable-for-microbes bodies through the gut, and infections drive many disease processes, lessening the risk of this happening has to be good news.

The upper gut – that is, the oesophagus, stomach and small intestine – should contain very low levels of microbes. It should be a near-sterile digesting gut for dealing with fat and protein. The lower gut – that is, large bowel – should be teeming with trillions of microbes which ferment vegetable fibre and resistant starches. Here we find two groups of fermenting microbes – approximately 10 per cent are oxygen tolerant (aerobes) and 90 per cent are oxygen intolerant (anaerobes).

Anaerobic microbes can be introduced into the gut only by a process that is not up for discussion in polite society, let alone in the standard cookbook (but then this book is far from standard). This is because anaerobic microbes are killed by oxygen and so cannot survive outside the gut. Normally we acquire these at birth from Mother and retain them for life by feeding them friendly prebiotics – that is, vegetable fibre, a staple of the PK diet. Modern high-carb diets and antibiotics can upset this delight-ful state of affairs. Faecal microbial therapy (a posh name for what my daughter has memorably named TT or 'turd transplant') is a logical and highly successful treatment for a variety of gut disorders, from ulcerative colitis to hospital-acquired *Clostridium difficile*. This is the only way I know of introducing anaerobic microbes into the gut.

The oxygen-tolerant microbes we can supply by fermenting nut, seed or soya milks to make yoghurts. We can also grow these microbes by making sauerkraut. There is still a huge amount of research needed to determine which microbes suit which person and which disease, so the following is simply a best guess which suits most – that includes me.

Kefir

The joy of using kefir is that one sachet of dried kefir (see page 137) can last a lifetime, making it a very inexpensive dish. The commonest cause of failure is not keeping the culture warm enough – remember, it ferments best in a hot, sweaty saddle bag and then in a human gut, both of which are at 37°C (98.6°F).

- Start off with one litre of long-life (that is, sterile) soya milk in a jug. (If you use coconut or hemp milk as a substrate, because these are so low in carbohydrate, I suggest adding a spoonful of sugar to give the kefir something to ferment.)
- Add a sachet of kefir (or pinch some live culture from a friend!).
- Keep in a warm place close to 37°C (98.6°F). You may need to use a yoghurt maker to achieve this. Within 18 hours it should have turned into a semi-solid, junket-like consistency, with some clear 'whey' on the surface. I drink this.
- Do not expect kefir to look like commercial yoghurt – often this has been thickened artificially.
- Once fermented, keep the culture in the fridge, where it will ferment further but more slowly. This slower fermentation seems to improve the texture and flavour.
- Kefir can be used at once as a substitute in any situation where you would previously have used cream or custard.

I use a cup of kefir daily to swallow my daily supplements; this means at least one cupful is used every day and stops me forgetting about the culture lurking in my fridge. If you do forget, or leave it for a week on holiday, it may acquire a slightly pink membranous crust. Scrape this off and use what is underneath to get another batch going. I have tried eating this crust – it is a bit sharp on the palate but did me no harm!

Once the jug is nearly empty, add another litre of soya or nut milk, stir it in (using a wooden or plastic spoon as kefir does not like contact with metal), keep it at room temperature and away you go again. I don't even bother to wash up the jug – the slightly hard yellow bits on the edge I just stir in to restart the brew. This way a sachet of kefir lasts for life, as I said. Furthermore, adding supplements to the brew is a good way of sneaking them into the diet of a recalcitrant and disbelieving family. It seems to be a very British thing to not want to take supplements – because these nutritional flat-earthers confidently state that, of course, 'Nothing is the matter with me and I eat a balanced diet.' I add a capsule of multivitamins together with a pinch of sunshine salt. Indeed, it is possible these nutrients may be incorporated into the bacteria and which thereby enhance their bioavailability.

Added extras: Add a lump of creamed coconut to the ferment; this further feeds the kefir, imparting a delicious coconut flavour, and thickens the culture.

Thick yoghurt

To make a lovely thick yoghurt:
- Take 500 ml of fermented kefir
- Add ½ cupful of warm, runny coconut oil
- ½ teaspoon of sunflower lecithin
- Whizz it all up in a Nutribullet, or equivalent
- Put in the fridge – it sets to a delicious 'gloop'.

Porridge
To make a thick porridge:
- Add to the kefir a handful of ground-up nuts or seeds, such as almond, linseed, chia, sunflower, poppy and/or pumpkin
- These absorb the fluid and turn the mix into a thick gloop. Jolly good!

Sauerkraut

Sauerkraut originally evolved to sustain us through the winter when vegetables would otherwise be unavailable and vitamins in poor supply. Again, the process of fermentation preserves not just the vegetable, but also us.

My horses are equally appreciative of fermented vegetables. My local farmer cuts grass for me and ferments it in polythene wraps – this is what is called silage, or haylage. My horses prefer this to hay – indeed it smells so good I fancy it myself! The pigs love it too.

Sauerkraut is amazingly easy to make – so easy that not only can I make it, but so have many other peoples. Some attention to detail is important – particularly oxygen and temperature. The same technique is used to make kimchi in Korea (cabbage, radish, scallion, cucumber), atchara in the Philippines (from papaya), curtido in Central America (cabbage, carrot, onion, oregano), dill pickles (cucumber), kiseil kupus in Serbia and kuceno in Bulgaria (cabbage).

In South Korea, kimchi is eaten at breakfast, lunch and dinner, with the average South Korean eating about 150-200 grams per day in winter, and 50-100 grams in summer. Eating alone is something of a taboo in South Korea and so this tradition of eating kimchi is passed down from generation to generation, with women being slightly larger consumers. The Japanese too have fermented foods as an essential part of their daily diet. Two condiments, for example, are miso (fermented soybean paste) and soy sauce. Also, natto, made of fermented soybeans, is eaten as a standard breakfast food. Japan has the highest life expectancy in the world – 83.7 years – and South Korean women have the third highest life expectancy among women at 85.5 years.[4]

Table 15: Making sauerkraut

Choose your ingredients and weigh the vegetables…	…This is to get the proportion of salt correct
Do not wash the vegetables…	…or you lose the friendly bacteria that are naturally present and essential for the fermentation
Cabbage is the main ingredient Cut out the solid core Cut the leaves into thin shreds no more than 5 mm wide	For a large batch use a food processor Add any other veg or fruit you fancy, such as red cabbage, carrot, beetroot, cooking apple Add spices such as caraway
Put the shreds into a large plastic bowl…	…not a metal container as the metal will contaminate the brew
Per 1 kilogram of cabbage plus other vegetables, add 20 grams of sunshine salt (for best flavour) or sea salt	The salt multitasks by pulling water out of the cabbage (by osmosis), hardening pectins for crunchiness, and inhibiting the growth of unfriendly bacteria (friendly lactobacilli are more tolerant of salt) so the sauerkraut can be stored for longer periods of time
Get your hands in to massage the mix and dissolve the salt. Mix it uniformly throughout and feel the cabbage wilting. Carry on until the mix feels very wet	It is really important to make sure the salt is distributed uniformly, otherwise the wrong microbes can flourish. My hands end up looking much cleaner by the time I have finished this job!

Stuff it all into a jar as full as you can, then press it down so the cabbage is covered with brine. Put on the lid, but do not put this on too tightly as the mix does produce some gas (see below)	I bought some sauerkraut online, then saved the jars for this job. The cabbage shreds must be under the surface of the saline. If you can't achieve this, add some more PK salt water. Shreds which are not covered by liquid may allow oxygen-loving bacteria and yeasts to ferment to produce 'off' flavours, scum and slime
Exclude as much air as you can because oxygen will spoil the ferment. You can help to do this by pouring a dollop of olive oil on the surface	This is an anaerobic (without oxygen) fermentation. Fermentation produces carbon dioxide which further helps exclude oxygen. The major microbe which ferments once oxygen is used up is *Lactobacillus plantarum* – this is an excellent anti-inflammatory microbe and of proven benefit in inflammatory bowel disease. Do not stir a ferment or you will introduce oxygen and wreck it. In this event, it may go brown (a sign that vitamin C has gone) or pink (a sign of yeast or mould), or produce a white film or slime
Put the lid on, not too tight OR get a special pot with an air lock	The fermentation will produce gas, so the lid must not be so tight that the pot explodes, but not so loose that oxygen can get in
	Check the pot of sauerkraut every so often – this is a great excuse to taste it. I often forget, but have yet to have a jar explode. This is by contrast with my childhood experiments making ginger beer illicitly in the airing cupboard upstairs – my mother was cross because her clean linen was spoiled and my father was cross because his bucket of mealworms were contaminated! (Note from Craig: My father would have been delighted by such an enterprise. His favourite drink was a 'Gunner' (see Wikipedia) – half ginger beer, half ginger ale with a dash of Angostura bitter.)
Temperature for fermenting is important	18-22°C (65-72°F) is ideal – that is, the highest shelf in my kitchen. Get a thermometer and measure this; it is surprisingly warm
Leave for at least four, ideally six, weeks	Do not put in the fridge until at least four weeks of fermentation at the above temperature have elapsed. Then screw the lids on tight to prevent any oxygen getting in. Storing in the fridge helps maintain the quality and this is essential once you start to eat it.

If you do not have the time, energy or inclination to make sauerkraut, then excellent organic and inexpensive ferments can be purchased through Goodness Direct (see page 137). Shamefully, since discovering this source, I now rarely make sauerkraut.

We leave this chapter with the wise words of Thomas Jefferson, in a letter to Thomas Cooper:

'I have wished to see chemistry applied to domestic objects… to fermentation…'

Thomas Jefferson, 13 April 1743 – 4 July 1826, was one of America's 'Founding Fathers', the principal author of the *Declaration of Independence* (1776) and second Vice President of the United States (1797–1801). Thomas Cooper (22 October 1759 – 11 May 1839) was an Anglo-American economist. He was described by Jefferson as 'one of the ablest men in America' and by John Adams as 'a learned ingenious scientific and talented madcap'.

13

Sunshine minerals – salts for the PK diet

Salt (sodium chloride – 'table salt') is much maligned nowadays but it is an essential part of our diet. Salt was recognised by the Ancients as absolutely necessary for our diet, and indeed the word 'salary' is derived from it (see Historical note below).

'Ye been the salt of the erthe and the savour'
The Summoner's Tale by Geoffrey Chaucer (circa 1343 – 25 October 1400) – This is the earliest publication of the phrase 'salt of the earth'' in the English language (circa 1386). (Chaucer is often called the 'Father of English literature', and is the first poet to have been buried in Poets' Corner in Westminster Abbey.)

Historical note 1: *'Salary' derives from the Latin 'salarium', which has the root 'sal', or 'salt'. There is much debate about the reasons for this; the most oft-quoted link is referenced from Pliny the Elder, who stated, as an aside in his* Natural History, *that 'In Rome... the soldier's pay was originally salt and the word salary derives from it...' Other newer sources state that Roman soldiers were paid in coins, and that the word 'salarium' is derived from the word 'sal' because a soldier may have been required by Army regulations to buy salt for his diet with some of said coins. Yet more sources state that the use of 'sal' as a root of 'salarium' derives from the price in coins that had to be paid by the Roman Empire to have soldiers conquer salt supplies and guard the Salt Roads (Via Salaria) that led to Rome. Even more intriguingly, some historians think that the word 'soldier' itself derives from the Latin 'sal dare' (to give salt), although I was taught that the word 'soldier' derives from the Latin for gold, 'solidus', with which soldiers were known to have been paid. Craig, via Mr Ferris, my Latin Master.*

Athletes are very aware of the importance of electrolytes (salts and minerals, which are actually the same thing). They are lost with intensive exercise through sweating, and in urine. Athletes are careful to replace sodium salt, but they forget the micro-minerals. The point here is that sweat is simply blood minus the solid bits (red cells, white cells, platelets and various proteins). All minerals are lost through it, and therefore a true electrolyte mix should include all minerals. Indeed, there are increasing reports of top athletes dropping dead with exercise. I suspect one unrecognised cause is acute magnesium deficiency. The link between sudden death and magnesium deficiency has long been known. For example, Eisenberg (1991) concludes that: 'A link between magnesium deficiency and sudden death is suggested by a substantial number of studies published over the past three decades.'[1]

With running, one loses about 10 milligrams of magnesium per mile through sweat and urine.[2] Calcium is necessary for heart muscle to contract; magnesium is necessary for heart muscle to relax. Exercise can induce an acute magnesium deficiency so that the heart stops in systole (the contraction phase of the cardiac cycle) – it does not have the magnesium needed for it to relax. In such cases, post mortem findings are normal because this is a functional problem, not an anatomical one.

Historical note 2: Magnesium is a 'paramagnetic' metal – that is, it is slightly attracted by a magnet. The Latin root is from 'Magnes', the Shepherd Boy, who was reported by Pliny the Elder to have been the accidental discoverer of magnetism. Pliny writes:

> *'Nicander is our authority that it [magnetite ore] was called Magnes, from the man who first discovered it on Mount Ida, and he is said to have found it when the nails of his shoes and the ferrule of his staff adhered to it, as he was pasturing his herds.'*

The said Nicander is of Colophon, a Greek poet, physician and grammarian. (Thanks again are due to Mr Ferris – it is a wonder we did any 'real' study! Craig)

Western diets are mineral deficient for several reasons:
1. We no longer recycle human sewage onto the fields. There is a net movement of minerals from the soil into plants, then into animals, then into us ... but now we throw what we excrete away. This means the mineral content of soils and foods has declined progressively since the 1950s. This is not my opinion (the decline in mineral content) but shown by government figures. Even organic food is micronutrient-deficient compared with the ideal, because failure to recycle also applies. The pattern is well illustrated by Figure 1, which shows mineral depletion in the United States since 1910.

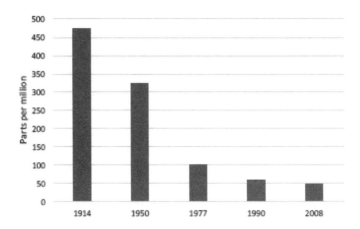

Figure 1: Soil mineral depletion in the United States since 1914 (Source: US Department of Agriculture and reproduced on myscienceacademy.org)

Please also see Anne-Marie Mayer's article in the *British Food Journal* (1997), which found that, in the 20 vegetables studied, there were statistically significant reductions in the levels of calcium, magnesium, copper and sodium of up to 25 per cent between 1930 and 1980 using geometric mean data.[3] It can only have worsened since then. Actual levels vary substantially, with some absolute drops of up to 94 per cent.

Here are some selected figures from Anne-Marie Mayer's article (percentage drops are shown in brackets in 'new' columns). Figures are expressed as mg/100 g of food type.

Food type	Ca old	Ca new	Mg old	Mg new	Cu old	Cu new	Na old	Na new
Brussels sprouts	28.7	26.0 (9%)	19.6	8.0 (59%)	0.05	0.02 (60%)	9.6	6.0 (37.5%)
Cabbage – winter	72.3	68.0 (6%)	16.8	6.0 (64%)	Reliable figure not available	0.02 (N/A)	28.4	3.0 (89%)

Celery	52.2	41.0 (21.5%)	9.6	5.0 (48%)	0.11	0.01 (91%)	137.0	60.0 (56%)
Onions	31.2	25.0 (20%)	7.6	4.0 (47%)	0.08	0.05 (37.5%)	10.2	3.0 (70.5%)
Parsley	325.00	200.00 (38%)	52.2	23.0 (56%)	0.52	0.03 (94%)	33.0	33.0 (Stable)

The old figures are from McCance and Widdowson (1960)[4] and the new from Holland et al (1991). [5]

Supporting these figures from the UK, we have this 2006 US comparison from the Nutrition Security Institute, which looked at summations of calcium (Ca), magnesium (Mg) and iron (Fe) in cabbage, lettuce, tomatoes and spinach and used four data points from Lindlahr (1914),[6] Hamaker (1982)[7] and the US Department of Agriculture (1963[8] and 1997[9]). Here is a graph of the results:

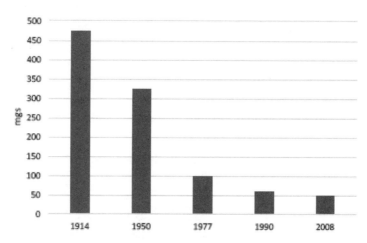

Figure 2: *Average mineral content of selected vegetables, 1914 to 1997 – sums of calcium, magnesium and iron in cabbage, lettuce, tomatoes and spinach.[6, 7, 8, 9]*

2. Modern Western diets, based on sugars and refined carbohydrates, may be rich in calories but are markedly deficient in micronutrients. Many micronutrients are stripped out in the refining process. I have yet to see normal tests of micronutrient status in anyone eating a Western diet who is not taking supplements.

3. We are no longer physically active and do not need to eat large amounts of food. Smaller amounts carry fewer micronutrients.
4. Our requirements for micronutrients are increasing because we live in an increasingly toxic world and we need micronutrients to detoxify.
5. Sunshine is considered to be a danger to health. Our sun phobia has resulted in widespread vitamin D deficiency and this is contributing to epidemics of osteoporosis, cancer and heart disease. Vitamin D greatly enhances the absorption of calcium and magnesium.

There is much more detail in our book *Sustainable Medicine*.

The PK diet goes some way to addressing these issues, but what I call 'sunshine salt' (which is described below) is an essential addition. Sunshine salt should be used in cooking and on food to substantially increase our intake of essential minerals. A further joy of sunshine salt is that a reluctant family can be effectively treated without resorting to coercion and bullying! (I was once caught out by my daughters when I experimented with B vitamins in bread – the loaf turned out bright yellow. I now sneak some into the kefir and they have yet to catch on. This is a test of whether they read my books!)

There is further reason to add sunshine salt – the requirement for minerals increases in people in ketosis. The bottom line is we should all be eating 5 grams (a rounded teaspoonful) of sunshine salt daily. This will supply you with the following:

Table 16: The mineral and vitamin content of sunshine salt

Essential mineral...	...in 5 grams of sunshine salt	For the man on the Clapham omnibus... (see footnote on page 101)	For the boffins, this mineral is essential for...
Sea salt (sodium chloride)	4 grams	Salt is much maligned nowadays but it is an essential part of our diet. Salt was recognised by the Ancients as essential for our diets and indeed the word 'salary' is derived from it.	...hydration, energy delivery, kidney function. (Sea salt contains other essential trace minerals in miniscule amounts, insufficient for normal human needs. So it must be reinforced with other minerals.)

Calcium chloride	60 milligrams	This amount is lower than the RDA (recommended daily allowance) but the extra vitamin D in sunshine salt greatly enhances its absorption	...muscle contraction (including heart muscle) and nerve conduction ...tough muscles, tendons and bones ...energy delivery in the body.
Magnesium (Mg) chloride	60 milligrams	This amount is lower than the RDA but the extra vitamin D in sunshine salt greatly enhances its absorption. Mg is 'Nature's tranquilliser'. Mg deficiency is pandemic in Western societies. Mg is essential for normal heart function; deficiency is a likely cause of sudden heart dysrhythmias.	...switching off the muscle contraction (so allowing the heart muscle to relax) and nerve excitation generated by calcium. ...energy delivery in the body (via mitochondria) ...as a co-factor for at least 300 different enzyme systems
Potassium chloride	40 milligrams	Potassium cannot be stored in the body so you need to consume this mineral daily.	...energy delivery mechanisms. All athletes should include potassium in their rehydration.
Zinc chloride	30 millgrams	Zinc deficiency is pandemic in Western societies. ZInc helps control blood sugar levels. ZInc is protective against heart disease and cancer. Vital for normal immunity Deficiency is associated with dyslexia.	...fighting infection ...detox in the liver ...DNA synthesis and repair ...the antioxidant superoxide dismutase ...protein synthesis ...hormone recognition.
Iron (ferric ammonium chloride)	15 milligrams	Lack of iron causes anaemia	...for haemoglobin which allows red cells to carry oxygen.
Boron (tetraborate)	2 milligrams	Highly protective against arthritis.	...normal calcium and magnesium metabolism.

Essential mineral…	…in 5 grams of sunshine salt	For the man on the Clapham omnibus…	For the boffins, this mineral is essential for…
Iodine (as potassium iodate)	1 milligram	Deficiency of iodine is extremely common (estimated to affect over 90% of Westerners). Thyroid disease is estimated to affect at least 20% of Westerners and one cause is iodine deficiency. Deficiency may manifest with breast pain, lumps and cysts.	…synthesis of thyroid hormones …synthesis of oxytocin (the love and empathy hormone – this may be a particular problem in autism.) …normal breast tissue.
Manganese (Mn)	1 milligram	Protects against damage to energy delivery mechanisms.	…manganese superoxide dismutase – the most important antioxidant within mitochondria.
Copper (Cu)	1 milligram	Copper provides links between fibres to make for tough connective tissue, muscle and bones. Deficiency can cause anaemia	…Zn/Cu superoxide dismutase - a vital antioxidant outside and inside all cells.
Molybdenum	200 micrograms	Helps detox in the liver – since we live in a toxic world this function is becoming increasingly important	….detox enzyme sulphite oxidase.
Selenium (Sn)	200 micrograms	Highly protective against cancer and heart disease. Gives connective tissue and bone their toughness and elasticity.	…glutathione peroxidase – a vital antioxidant.
Chromium	200 micrograms	Deficiency results in diabetes. Protective against heart disease.	…insulin.
Vitamin D3	5,000 iu	Deficiency is pandemic in Western sun-phobic society. D3 is highly protective against heart disease, cancer and autoimmunity. No toxicity has ever been seen in doses up to 10,000 iu daily.	…enhancing the absorption of calcium and magnesium and ensuring their deposition in bone. …normal immune function – it is an excellent anti-inflammatory and protective against many viral infections.

Vitamin B12	5,000 micrograms	Deficiency is pandemic in Westerners eating high carbohydrate diets. B12 is highly protective against heart disease, cancer and dementia. No toxicity. B12 poorly absorbed so high doses are essential. As we age and our bodies slow down, and our requirements for B12 increase.	…healing and repair, detoxification and protein synthesis, via the methylation cycle.

The above would be an excellent basis for a rehydrating mix for athletes or, indeed, people suffering from gastroenteritis. I would recommend using a rounded teaspoon (5 grams) of sunshine salt in 3 litres of water (approximately a 0.02 per cent solution). At this dilution one can hardly taste the salt but it will be doing a power of good. You can make your own sunshine salt following the proportions in the Table, or you can purchase it from my website (see page 137).

Legal note: The 'man on the Clapham omnibus' is a hypothetical ordinary and reasonable person, used by the courts in English law to decide whether a party has acted as a reasonable person would. If the 'man on the Clapham omnibus' would do a certain thing, or think it, then this would mean it is a reasonable action or thought. It was first put to use in the courts in a judgement by Sir Richard Henn Collins MR in 1903. He attributed it to Lord Bowen.

14

PK water

People eating Western diets are chronically dehydrated. Many realise this, but the answer is not to drink more water. Indeed, some of the worst nourished patients I have ever seen are those who think it is healthy to drink several litres of water a day. Whilst one can drink pure water, one cannot pee pure water – urine always contains all the minerals. Such excessive consumption washes precious minerals out of the body and worsens the dehydration.

To understand what we need so as to hydrate the body properly, we need to return to the elementary biology we learned in school and remember **osmosis**. This is the mechanism by which water is held within cells – 'a process by which molecules of a solvent (that is, water) tend to pass through a semipermeable membrane [such as a cell's outer membrane] from a less concentrated solution into a more concentrated one'. What this means is that for water to be held within a cell, firstly we need salts within that cell to 'pull' the water in and secondly we need fats/oils to create a good, semipermeable membrane.

Linguistic note: 'Osmosis' derives from the Greek osmos, ωσμος, 'a thrusting, a pushing', from the stem of othein, 'to thrust, to push'.

This means that any water that is consumed must be balanced up with essential salts (a rounded teaspoonful daily of sunshine salt (see page 94) – more if you exercise and sweat a lot) and an abundance of fats, including cholesterol.

On the PK diet, there are two vital types of fat in abundance. Firstly, there are the medium-chain fats, which act as fuels to power the body, from animals (lard), coconuts or palm oil. Secondly, we need long-chain fats (which are liquid oils at room temperature) for making good cell membranes. These fats (which include phospholipids) come from meat, fish, eggs, vegetables, nuts and seeds. Phospholipid oil molecules have a water-loving end and a fat-loving end which allows them naturally to line themselves up effortlessly into a lipid sandwich, with the water-loving ends facing out and the fatty tails facing in. This double-layer is the basic structure of all cell membranes; cholesterol is an essential part of the inside of these membranes. (Please see Appendix 1, page 109, for more detail on the biochemistry of these fats.)

We have the sensation of thirst for good reason – it tells us how much to drink. I do not see any point in drinking over and above thirst requirements. Having said that, many drinks are diuretic – they actually induce us to excrete more water so we should not be drinking them to quench thirst. Quench thirst with water or herbal teas (yes, I know some of these can be mildly diuretic too – dandelion and nettle are among the most extreme) – then use tea or coffee for pleasure and zip factor and go nowhere near fruit juices or 'juice drinks' and the like.

Drink the best water you can

Start with a good water filter
We live in an increasingly polluted world. Furthermore, mains water is treated with chlorine, chlorine dioxide and, worse, chloramine. Whilst these are helpful in disinfecting water, they inevitably leave harmful residues and taste disgusting. Having become accustomed to spring water, my horses will not drink mains water! (They will not eat a supermarket apple either.) Water filters are an essential part of any PK kitchen and good ones (check specifications) are effective at removing chlorine and heavy metals.

Avoiding fluoride
However, if your water is fluoridated, a simple water filter won't do. This is because these filters do not remove fluoride. Fluoride is a nasty, toxic element, ostensibly added to prevent tooth decay, but really in order to dispose of a toxic by-product of industry. It is an endocrine disruptor (that means it messes up our production of hormones, especially thyroxin) and may well explain our current epidemic of hypothyroidism (underactive thyroid). It is also a probable carcinogen (especially related to bone cancer); it is deposited in and weakens bone (increasing fracture risk) and it readily combines with aluminium to encourage deposition of both in the brain, with dementia resulting. The current fashion for fluoride in water, dentistry and toothpaste is a health disaster.

No filter gets rid of fluoride completely. You will have to shop around to find one that suits. Many of the toxicities associated with fluoride result because iodine deficiency is pandemic, so using sunshine salt will help protect against any residual fluoride.

Bottled water
If you are drinking bottled water rather than filtering, use either glass or as large a plastic container as you can. Glass is, of course, inconvenient and heavy. However, for some of my patients who are very sensitive, water in glass bottles is the only water they can drink. Most plastics contain softeners, such as bisphenol A (BPA), which

inevitably contaminate water. This is why you should avoid small bottles and also not let them get warm. When left in heat, levels of BPA increase (see the article 'Don't drink the (warm) water left in a plastic bottle UF/IFAS study says'[1] and the original study on which it is based.[2]). A large container reduces the ratio of surface area to volume of water and so reduces the potential for contamination.

Drink the best quality water that you can, but be aware that though it may be called 'mineral water' the low levels in all bottled waters will not provide an alternative to sunshine salt.

I am extremely fortunate to have several springs behind my house for water. If I were not so blessed, then for drinking and cooking purposes I would install a rainwater harvesting system and use an ultraviolet light to disinfect it. (There is a high rainfall in my part of Wales!)

Though plain water is best, I love sparkling water and for this I suggest purchasing a soda stream to carbonate water.

Conclusion

Craig leaves you with a quotation that was ancient even during the times of Pliny the Elder, who himself quoted it. The fact that the first half of this quote is the most remembered perhaps is a reflection of the nature of mankind itself ...

'In vino veritas, in aqua sanitas' – *in wine there is truth, in water there is health.*

'But make sure it is the right kind of aqua!' – Dr Sarah Myhill.

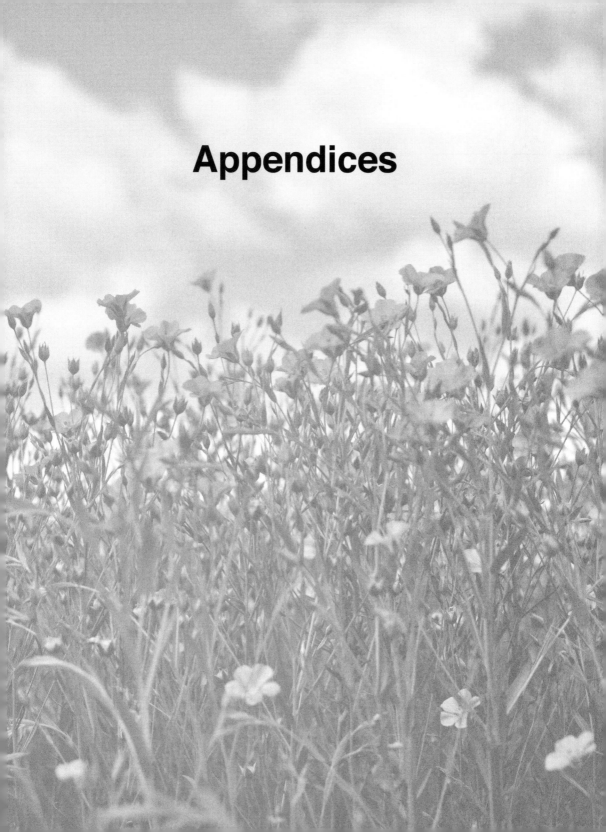

Appendices

Appendix 1
Good fats and bad fats

Broadly speaking, we have two types of fat – medium-chain fats and long-chain fats. (See Chapter 3 for detail on short-chain fatty acids, which are not included here, and also our book *Prevent and Cure Diabetes*.) The medium-chain fats, such as lard, butter, coconut fat and chocolate fat, are used as fuels to power the body. These are 'saturated fats'. For the biochemists, in a saturated fat, every carbon atom is saturated either with another carbon or a hydrogen atom. This renders the fat stiff and stable, so, when heated (which shakes things up) it retains its normal shape. These stiff fats are solid at room temperature.

Generally speaking, medium-chain fat molecules consist of between eight and 14 carbon atoms, whilst long-chain fat molecules have more than 14 carbon atoms and short-chain fat molecules fewer than eight. To describe one fat, for example, approximately 50 per cent of the fat content of coconut fat is made up of lauric acid. Lauric acid has a melting point 43.8°C (110.84°F) and so is solid at room temperature. Its molecules consist of 12 carbon atoms and it is therefore a medium-chain fat. In addition, lauric acid is saturated, and so, being a medium-chain saturated fat, fits the bill as being one of the fats that retain their normal shape when heated, because of its stiffness and stability. If you will forgive the O level lesson (I am now showing my age!), Figure 3 is a diagram of lauric acid – you will see the 12 carbon atoms and that all the bonds are 'saturated'.

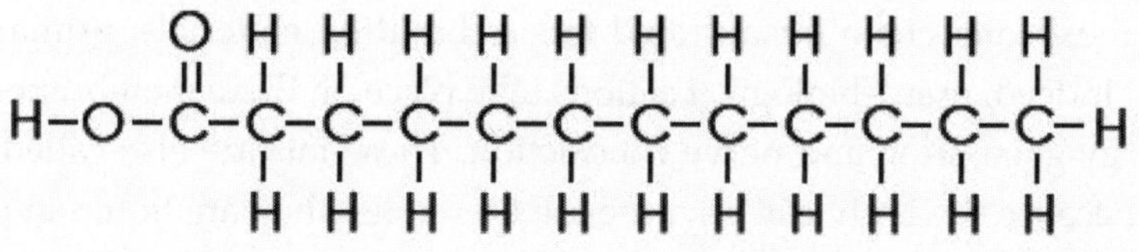

Figure 3: A lauric acid molecule

The second type of fat is a long-chain unsaturated fat. The occasional hydrogen atom is 'missing' and so we get a double carbon bond instead. If we have one double carbon bond, then we call this fat 'mono-unsaturated' (this includes olive oil) and if we have more than one double carbon bond, we call this fat 'poly-unsaturated'. (This includes most nut, seed, vegetable and fish oils). This double carbon bond 'kinks' the molecule and the molecule is named according to where the kink is – for example, an omega-3 fat has its kink at the third carbon atom, an omega-6 at the sixth and an omega-9 at the ninth. Figure 4 shows what this kinking may look like diagrammatically.

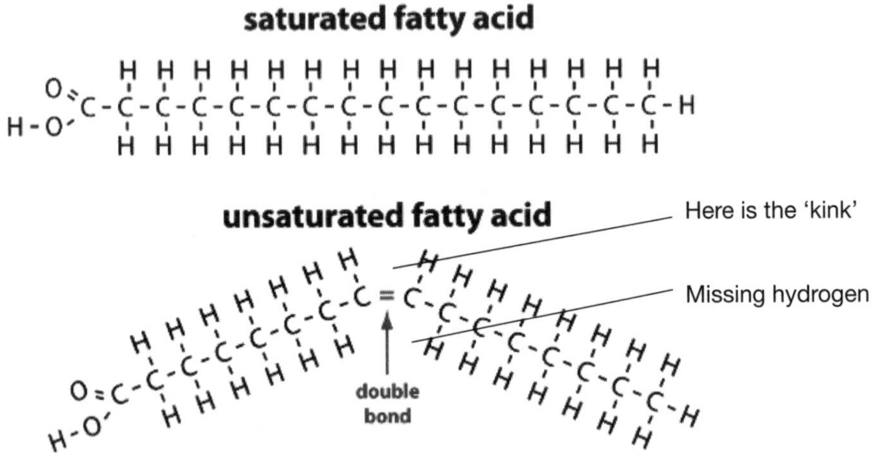

saturated fatty acid

unsaturated fatty acid

Figure 4: *The difference between a saturated and an unsaturated fat molecule showing the double bond and 'kink' that makes an unsaturated fat unstable. This unsaturated fat is a 'mono-unsaturated fat' because it has only one double-bond/kink in its carbon chain*

We use these long-chain unsaturated fats as building materials, primarily in cell membranes. Indeed, many biological actions take place on these membranes – actions such as energy generation and nerve conduction. These fats are also called 'essential fatty acids' because the body can't synthesise these oils (they are liquid at room temperature) for itself – they have to be eaten.

Trans-fats

You may be aware that when unsaturated fats, which are inherently less stable than saturated, are heated they can be turned into unnatural 'trans-fats' that are not suitable for human consumption. In Nature, kinks in unsaturated fats such as are shown in Figure 4 are all so-called 'left-handed' (this relates to their shape) and are called 'cis-fats'. They fit our biochemistry perfectly. Problems arise when these fats are heated or 'hydrogenated' (to create 'spreads' such as margarine) and they flip into a 'right-handed' version – these are trans-fats. Just as a right hand will not fit into a left-hand glove, so trans-fats do not fit our biochemistry, and so they clog up systems and are highly damaging. Figure 5 shows the problem; the trans-fat is not the same shape as the cis-fat and so will not fit with our biochemistry.

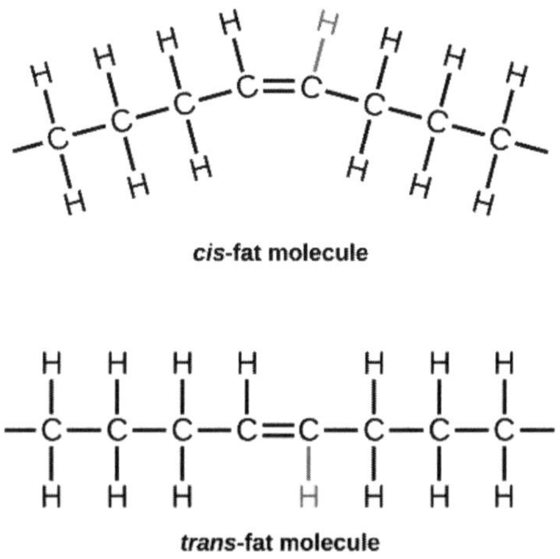

cis-fat molecule

trans-fat molecule

Figure 5: *Comparison of the structure of a natural cis-fat and that of a trans-fat created by over-heating or hydrogenation*

It follows that the rules of the game are:
- Do not eat hydrogenated fats (as in margarine and other 'spreads') – if the fat has been hydrogenated, then the resulting trans-fat will not fit with your biochemistry
- Cook with saturated fats such as lard (any animal fat), butter or coconut oil – these fats retain their shape after cooking

- Use cold-pressed oils (as opposed to fats, which are solid) at room temperature – do not cook with them. If they are liquid at room temperature they are relatively unstable and therefore susceptible to damage. As I have said, cooking will change these oils so they will no longer fit with our biochemistry.

Appendix 2
Essential equipment for the PK kitchen

The golden rule is: keep it simple, quick and easy.

The main aim of equipment is to reduce work and washing up. I have as little equipment as I can get away with, so it is all immediately to hand – for example, my Nutribullet lives on the worktop permanently plugged in as I use it daily for PK bread, PK ice cream, soups and smoothies.

Dishwashers wash and rinse plates far more effectively than humans. I recommend two half -size dishwashers, one for the dirty loading, one clean for current use. That way you do not waste time or energy unloading and stashing kitchen implements. Crocks and cutlery live permanently in the dishwasher. A canine pre-wash improves the end result since the crusty bits which stick to oven dishes clearly taste awfully good. (Do use relatively ecological dishwasher tablets such as Ecover rather than strong chemicals that are bad for you as a residue and for the environment.)

I have a plastic jug in which kefir resides permanently, albeit alternating between warm kitchen for fermenting and fridge for keeping. It is washed up very occasionally – my record is two months of no washing up.

The slow-cooker for bones again is permanently on with no washing up – the heat prevents infection. Bones go in and out, cooking vegetable water goes in, so does sunshine salt and delicious stock (aka broth) results.

Cooking equipment must be safe

We all remember the phase when we threw out our aluminium cooking pans and replaced them with stainless steel. Miserably, stainless steel is 14 per cent nickel. Nickel is a major sensitising metal for switching on allergy, and is a known carcinogen.

I am in the throes of auditing all the toxicity tests that I do. These include 'DNA adducts'. This is a test for substances stuck on to DNA. Of course there should be nothing stuck to our DNA – it should be pristine. Nickel is one of the commonest adducts so do not use stainless steel cookware. The next most frequent adducts are dyes (from food and hair colourants) and flame retardants from soft furnishings.

Non-stick is worse – it releases perfluoro-octanic acid with all the problems associated with fluoride (see page 105).

Copper cookware is not too bad, but acidic foods will leach copper out freely.

So what is safe to use? For cooking use pots and pans made from cast iron, pyrex, enamel, ceramic or stone. For mixing I use pottery or hard ancient plastic. (Mine have had 60 years to give off their gases… yes, yes they are Mother's hand-me-downs.)

Appendix 3
Carb values for vegetables, salads, fruits, berries, nuts and seeds

'He who does not mind his belly, will hardly mind anything else.'
Samuel Johnson (1709-1784) British author of the first English language dictionary.

This Appendix consists of lists of the 'net' (see below) carbohydrate content of vegetables and salads, fruits and berries, nuts and seeds, and grains and pulses. It is far from exhaustive. The carbohydrate values are for the most part taken from the relevant USDA (United States Department of Agriculture) Database entries. For those who are interested, please see details of Release 28 of the USDA National Nutrient Database for Standard.[1] You may find variations on the internet, or elsewhere, but these figures are a very good guide.

I have separated each list into:
- green – up to 5 grams of carbs per 100 grams or less than 5 per cent carb. These can be eaten pretty much *ad lib* (or you would have to eat over 500 grams to start to run into problems. Even greedy me can't manage that.)
- amber – 5-10 grams of carbs per 100 grams or more than 5 per cent but less than 10 per cent carb. Measure these out carefully.
- red – more than 10 grams of carbs per 100 grams or more than 10 per cent carb. These must be very, very carefully rationed. It is safest to avoid them altogether as they tend to switch on addictive eating. They should be for occasional use only as it is so easy to eat too much.

For guidance I prefer to use net carbs (sugars and starches, with fibre excluded) on the grounds that fibre is fermented into short-chain fatty acids in the large bowel and these are a good source of alternative, non-carb energy (see Chapters 3 and 5 and also our book *Prevent & Cure Diabetes*). Linseed is such a great food (see Chapter 2, PK

115

bread, page 15) because, although 100 grams of it contains 29 grams of total carbs, 27 grams are made up of fibre and so there are just 2 grams of starch and sugar.

Always look at the labels on 'bought foods'. These will detail the carbohydrate content, which can be very helpful. The carbohydrate values given on labels are normally total carbs which include all starches, sugars and soluble fibre. Try to tease out the net carb figure if you can by subtracting the fibre from 'total carbs'. In the following lists, the net carb content in grams per 100 grams of food-type is included next to the food type.

Note: Protein eaten in excess can be converted into sugars. A rule of thumb is to allow 0.7 to 0.9 grams (g) of protein per pound (0.45 kg) of lean body mass. Remember, the PK diet is *not* a high-protein diet. It is a high-fat, high-fibre diet.

Food	Protein content in g per 100 g	On the plate looks like... approx
Eggs	13	One egg
Beef	26	A medium beef burger
Pork	31	Small pork chop
Bacon	Up to 39 depending on how fat! One slice 8 g	
Lamb	26	One lamb chop
Chicken, duck	20	Whole breast, or Whole leg
Fish, fresh	29	A good chunk!
Prawns	25	A prawn 'cocktail' starter

So, for example, I weigh 140 lb (63 kg) which means my lean body is about 100 lb (45 kg). You can calculate this at

https://www.calculator.net/lean-body-mass-calculator.html

This means I can eat 80 g of protein a day without reducing my carb ration. For me this amounts to:

- Breakfast: 2 eggs (26 g), 2 rashers bacon (16 g) (My bacon is very fat)
- Supper: tinned fish starter (8 g), pork chop (30 g)

If you exceed the protein limit then this should be deducted from the daily carb ration on the approximate basis that one gram of protein can be converted to one gram of carb.

Green

As I've said, these have up to 5 grams of net carb per 100 grams of the food – that is, they are less than 5 per cent carb.

Vegetables	Salads	Nuts, nut butters and seeds	Fruits for pudding	Grains and pulses	Miscellaneous
Pak choi – 1.2 Curly kale – 1.3 Spinach – 1.4 Asparagus – 1.8 Collards – 2.0 Marrow-2.0 Courgette (zucchini) – 2.1 Swiss chard – 2.1 Mushrooms – 2.3 Tomatoes – 2.7 Bamboo shoots – 2.8 Aubergine (eggplant) – 3.0 Cauliflower – 3.0 Cabbage – 3.5 Green beans – 3.6 Okra – 3.8 Fennel – 3.9 Turnip –4.2 Broccoli – 4.4 Spring onions – 4.4 Cress – 4.9	Alfalfa sprouts –0.2 Endive – 0.3 Chicory – 0.7 Watercress – 0.8 Celery – 1.4 Lettuce, romaine – 1.2 Lettuce – 1.6 Radish – 1.8 Chives – 2 Avocado – 2 Tomato – 2.7 Olives 3.8 Cucumber – 3.1	Hemp seed – 2.8 Brazil nuts – 4.0 Pecans – 4.0	Rhubarb – 2.7	Linseed (aka Flax seed) – 2.0 – which is why the PK bread is so good!	Vinegars – 0 Sunflower lecithin – 0 Tofu – 1.0 Quorn – 1.0 Coconut kefir – 3.8 Soy sauce – 4.1

Amber

As explained above, these contain 5-10 grams of net carbs per 100 grams – that is, they are more than 5 per cent but less than 10 per cent net carb.

Vegetables	Salads	Nuts, nut butters and seeds	Fruits for pudding	Grains and pulses	Miscellaneous
Brussels sprouts – 5.2 Squash spaghetti – 5.5 Artichoke (globe) -6.0 Pumpkin – 6.5 Corn, baby sweetcorn – 6.5 Swede – 6.7 Celeriac – 7.2 Beetroot – 7.2 Carrots – 7.2 Onions – 7.3	Capsicum pepper – 7.5	Coconut – 6 Almond – 6.0 Macadamia nuts – 6.0 Walnuts – 7.0 Peanuts – 7.0 Hazelnuts – 7.0 Chia seeds – 8.0 Poppy seeds – 8.0 Tiger nuts – 9.0 Pine nuts – 9.3	Raspberry – 5.0 Blackberry – 5.0 Gooseberry – 5.7 Strawberry – 6.0 Lemon – 6.2 Cranberry – 6.4 Black/Redcurrants – 6.6 Cantaloupe – 7.2 Water melon – 7.6 Lime – 8.2 Mulberry – 8.3 Peach – 8.5 Apricot – 9.0 Nectarine – 9.3 Grapefruit – 9.4 Plum – 9.6 Orange – 9.6	Peas – 9.0	Hummus – 8.0

Red

These foods contain more than 10 grams of net carbs per 100 grams – that is, are more than 10 per cent net carbs.

Vegetables	Salads	Nuts, nut butters and seeds	Fruits	Grains and pulses	Miscellaneous
Squash, butternut – 10.0 Leeks – 12 Lentils – 12 Parsnip – 13.1 Shallots – 13.8 Potatoes – 14.8 Artichokes (Jerusalem) – 15 Sweet potato – 28.0		Almonds – 10.0 Sesame seeds – 11.0 Sunflower seeds – 11.0 Psyllium husks – 11.1 Tahini (sesame seed butter) – 11.5 Pumpkin seed butter – 12.0 Coriander seed – 12.0 Caraway – 12.0 Peanut butter – 14.0 Chestnut butter – 16.5 Almond butter – 17.5 Pistachios – 18.0 Pomegranate seeds – 18.7 Cashew butter – 26.0 Chestnuts – 26.0 Cashews – 26.7 Cumin seeds – 35.0 Pumpkin seeds – 36.0 Hazelnut butter – 57.0	Clementine – 10.3 Cherry – 10.4 Elderberry – 11.0 Guava – 11.0 Satsuma – 11.2 Blueberry – 11.3 Apple – 11.3 Pineapple – 11.6 Pear – 11.9 Kiwi – 12.0 Passionfruit – 13.0 Quince – 13.1 Mango –13.4 Pomegranate – 15.0 Grapes – 16.1 Banana – 20.4	Oats 10.3 Quinoa – 17 Brown rice – 21 Kidney beans – 35 Haricot beans (as in baked beans) – 36 (My most hated breakfast cereals, which must be nameless, like 'frosted' rice, are 89% carb)	100% dark chocolate – 14.0 Cacao powder – 16.5 85% dark chocolate – 22.5 Carob – 23.5 Cocoa powder – 25.0 Baking powder – 27.8

Foods that can be eaten *ad lib*

You can eat the following in any quantity because they contain zero carbs:
- Fats that are safe to cook with:
    ◊ Animal fats: lard, dripping, butter, goose fat
    ◊ Vegetable fats: coconut oil, palm oil, cocoa fat
- Fats you must not cook with:
    ◊ Fish oils
    ◊ Vegetable, nut and seed oils: olive, hemp, rape, sunflower, grapeseed, peanut, corn etc
- Sauerkraut

Proteins such as meat, eggs, fish and shellfish contain no carbs BUT, if eaten in excess (as described on page 116), can be converted by the body into sugars.

Foods that should form no part of the PK diet

Very high carb foods should form no part of a PK diet and should be avoided:
- Grains: wheat, corn, barley, rice, oats, quinoa
- Pulses: chick peas, baked beans, kidney beans, soya beans
- Fruits: apples, bananas, pears, oranges, pineapple, mango, papaya, grapes, melon (Yes, I know they are delicious but they are all a bag of sugar)
- Dried fruits: dates, figs, sultanas, raisins, goji berries, cranberries, apricots, prunes (However, I admit I use these in tiny amounts to give a hint of sweetness to PK buns – I told you I was no paragon!)
- Fruit juices and fruit smoothies
- Sweet drinks, pop, sports and 'energy' drinks
- Honey, sugars, treacle
- Sweeteners – natural or artificial
- Milk, cream, cheese, yoghurt (from cow, buffalo, goat or sheep)

Appendix 4
Nutritional supplements for the PK diet

Primitive man (or woman!) did not require nutritional supplements. Modern Western man eating even a PK diet does, for the following obvious and logical reasons:

- There is now a one-way movement of minerals from the soil, to plants, animals and humans. We no longer recycle these minerals back to the land and therefore there is a net depletion of minerals from the soil and ultimately from food. Moreover, if plants do not have minerals, then they cannot make the vitamins and essential fatty acids that are vital for animal and human life.
- Most of our crops, including those which are used to feed farm animals, are annual crops, so that only the upper few inches of soil are exploited.
- This nutritious topsoil is being rapidly depleted by modern farming techniques.
- The mineral deficiencies which result increase the need for pesticides and herbicides. These toxic chemicals create further problems downstream because:
  a) Many pesticides, such as glyphosate, work by chelating minerals in soil, thereby reducing mineral availability to plants, thus further increasing the need for pesticides.
  b) The use of nitrogen fertilizers and pesticides reduces the humus content (the mycorrhiza – a symbiotic association composed of fungus and roots of a vascular plant) of soil and therefore plants will not absorb minerals properly, thus further increasing the need for pesticides.
  c) Pesticides increase the toxic load in food; these toxins require more micronutrients for the body to detoxify and excrete them.
- Genetically modified crops – genetic modification is largely done to develop pesticide-resistant strains rather than for improving micronutrient density. More pesticide is therefore used, exacerbating the above problems.
- Crops may be bred or genetically modified for their appearance or keeping qualities, at the expense of good micronutrient content.

- Modern man does not exercise as much as primitive man – consequently he needs to eat less food, which means fewer micronutrients. Even recently, actual calorie consumption has fallen – in Britain, we eat 600 fewer calories daily than 30 years ago.
- Many modern foods (and this applies more to people who do not eat PK) deplete nutrients directly. Refined carbohydrates are the best example.

For further reading please see the Nutrition Security Institute's White Paper: Human Health, the Nutritional Quality of Harvested Food and Sustainable Farming Systems[1] which quotes US Senate Document #264 (published in 1936) that: 'The alarming fact is that foods – fruits, vegetables and grains – now being raised on millions of acres of land that no longer contains enough of certain needed nutrients, are starving us – no matter how much we eat of them' and concludes (in 2006): 'Our food system is rapidly losing its ability to produce food with nutrient levels adequate to maintain the health of our families.'

What is the minimum we can get away with?

The problem is that many of us hate taking supplements. I find any such suggestion is met with the classic nutritional Flat-Earther's comment, 'Well, I am eating a healthy balanced diet.' (The speaker is usually a man!) So what is the absolute minimum that we can get away with? The PK diet that includes PK salt will provide all the necessary minerals, essential fatty acids and vitamin D. So I suggest in addition:

- **Mornings:** Take a good multivitamin (I have tried disguising these in food and so far failed miserably). Put the pot of multivits on the breakfast table – then you will remember.
- **Evenings:** Take vitamin C – at least 2 grams, possibly more. Leave the pot of vitamin C next to the toothbrush and fluoride-free toothpaste – then you will remember.

Note on vitamin C: It is humans, fruit bats and guinea pigs that cannot make their own vitamin C. My dog Nancy does not get scurvy whatever her diet because she can make her own vitamin C. The RDA (recommended dietary allowance) for vitamin C in humans is 30 milligrams; this may stop you getting scurvy but it is far too low for optimal health. One report states a 70 kilo (155 lb) goat makes 13,000 milligrams (13 grams or 0.46 ounces) of vitamin C daily. Linus Pauling, the only person to win two unshared Nobel prizes, advocated 10 grams daily. However, many people would get diarrhoea at this dose. I take 4 grams at night every day, but much more at the first symptom of a cough or cold. (For much more detail see our books *Sustainable Medicine* and *The Natural Treatment of Infection: Life is an Arms Race*.)

Taking supplements can be a bore – you must, as with so many things, have the will to do it, knowing that it will make a positive difference:

> *'Our bodies are our gardens, to the which our wills are gardeners'*
> *Othello* Act 1 Scene 3, William Shakespeare, April 1564 – 23 April 1616

Appendix 5

Seven-day meal plan for the severely disabled and/or for those people who are otherwise challenged by energy/time and/or inclination

The following seven-day meal plan (repeated from our book *Prevent and Cure Diabetes*) is not intended to be prescriptive (everybody is different, as we've said). Primarily, it is for the severely disabled and/or for those people who are otherwise challenged by energy/time and/or inclination. It follows on from Chapter 2. For some people it may help to give them an idea of how they might initially approach a paleo-ketogenic way of eating so that they can easily get started. Don't stick to it in the long term or you will get bored and that is often a cause of failure.

This plan demonstrates that the paleo-ketogenic diet can be followed even if the individual is suffering severe disability. The idea is to provide a list of meal and food suggestions that require no preparation or cooking. In essence, this can be a temporary measure until you can cook more independently or until you have more time, and so don't think that this will have to be your diet forever. In fact, following this diet will give you more energy so that you become more able to cook independently and enjoy the other meals as described in this book.

Some people will need to go through this initial 'no cooking and no preparation' stage before they are able to move on to the delicious recipes found in the rest of the book, whereas some people will be able to 'skip' straight to those more appealing recipes without first going through this 'no cooking and no preparation' stage. But the meal ideas in this Appendix may be useful for all, if a 'quick fix' PK meal is needed at any time.

Please note, when following the plan below, that for breakfasts, where there is advice to mix seeds with Coyo or Alpro yoghurt, different people will have different tastes as to how 'thick' they would like this to be. Please adjust the amount of seeds you mix in to your own taste, but do make sure that you eat all the seeds.

Day 1: Ketogenic meal suggestions

Breakfast: Day 1

Food	Protein (grams)	Carbohydate (grams)	Calories (kCal)
Coyo natural yoghurt (125 grams)	4.0	0.6	228
Mix in 100 grams of chia seeds	17.0	8.0	486
1 slice of PK bread (see page 21) (Approx. amounts)	5.0	0.5	125
With some macadamia nut butter spread on this slice (say, 10 grams)	2.0	1.35	70
Totals	28.0	10.45	909

Lunch: Day 1

Food	Protein (grams)	Carbohydrate (grams)	Calories (kCal)
Tinned mackerel in basil and tomato sauce (120 grams)	15.36	6.84	158
Two avocados (say, 200 grams)	4.0	4.0	320
Frozen berries from the freezer – 50 grams of blueberries	0.3	6.7	30
Total	19.66	17.54	508

Mid-afternoon snack: Day 1 (But try to avoid snacking)

Food	Protein (grams)	Carbohydrate (grams)	Calories (kCal)
Salami – Serious Pig snacking (50 grams) (see page 18)	16.0	0.0	211
Total	16.0	0.0	211

Supper: Day 1

Food	Protein (grams)	Carbohydrate (grams)	Calories (kCal)
Tinned tuna in spring water (120 grams)	32.4	Trace	135
50 grams each of tomato,	0.45	1.35	9
cucumber,	0.7	0.8	8
lettuce	0.35	1.65	8
Dollop mayonnaise (10 grams) (see Recipes, page 59)	0.1	Trace	68
Pine nuts (20 grams)	2.8	1.9	135
Total	36.8	5.7	363

Drinks: Day 1

Sparkling water as necessary; maximum of three cups of tea/coffee. (All negligible for carbs.)

Totals for Day 1

> **Calories – 1991 kCal**
> **Carbs – 33.69 grams**
> **Protein – 100.46 grams**

Day 2: Ketogenic meal suggestions

Breakfast: Day 2

Food	Protein (grams)	Carbohydrate (grams)	Calories (kCal)
Alpro vanilla yoghurt (200 grams)	7.4	19.0	150
Mix in 100 grams of hemp seeds	24.0	2.8	455
1 slice of PK bread (see page 21) (Approx. amounts)	5.0	0.5	125
With some hazelnut nut butter spread on this slice (say, 10 grams)	1.3	1.6	63
Totals	37.7	23.9	793

Lunch: Day 2

Food	Protein (grams)	Carbohydrate (grams)	Calories (kCal)
Chopped pork (200 gram tin)	33.8	1.2	414
50 grams each of tomato,	0.45	1.35	9
cucumber,	0.7	0.8	8
lettuce	0.35	1.65	8
Frozen berries from freezer – 50 grams of strawberries	0.35	3.0	17
Total	35.65	8.0	456

Mid-afternoon snack: Day 2 (But try to avoid snacking)

Food	Protein (grams)	Carbohydrate (grams)	Calories (kCal)
One half bar Green and Black's 85% chocolate	4.7	11.25	315
Total	4.7	11.25	315

Supper: Day 2

Food	Protein (grams)	Carbohydrate (grams)	Calories (kCal)
Tinned grilled sardines (120 grams)	27.36	0.0	237
One avocado (say 100 grams)	2.0	2.0	160
Total	29.36	2.0	397

Drinks: Day 2

Sparkling water as necessary; maximum of three cups of tea / coffee. (All negligible for carbs.)

Totals: Day 2

Calories – 1961 kCal

Carbs – 45.15 grams

Protein – 107.41 grams

Day 3: Ketogenic meal suggestions

Breakfast: Day 3

Food	Protein (grams)	Carbohydrate (grams)	Calories (kCal)
Coyo chocolate coconut yoghurt (125 grams)	2.9	4.9	245
Mix in 50 grams of pumpkin seeds	9.5	18.0	223
1 slice of PK bread (see page 21) (Approx. amounts)	5.0	0.5	125
With some peanut nut butter spread on this slice (say, 10 grams)	2.6	1.7	60
Pine nuts (20 grams)	2.8	1.9	135
Totals	22.8	27.0	788

Lunch: Day 3

Food	Protein (grams)	Carbohydrate (grams)	Calories (kCal)
Tinned gammon (200 grams)	36.0	2.6	200
Sauerkraut (pot 100 grams)	0.7	1.4	19
Alpro soya yoghurt, plain (150 grams)	6.0	3.15	75
Almonds (30 grams)	6.3	3.0	172
Total	49.0	10.15	466

Mid-afternoon snack (but try to avoid snacking)

Food	Protein (grams)	Carbohydrate (grams)	Calories (kCal)
Pecans (50 grams)	4.5	2.0	345
Total	4.5	2.0	345

Supper: Day 3

Food	Protein (grams)	Carbohydrate (grams)	Calories (kCal)
Corned beef (125 gram tin)	31.0	1.38	282
50 grams each of tomato,	0.45	1.35	9
cucumber,	0.7	0.8	8
lettuce	0.35	1.65	8
Dollop mayonnaise (10 grams) (see page 59)	0.1	Trace	68
Total	32.6	5.18	375

Drinks: Day 3

Sparkling water as necessary; maximum of three cups of tea/coffee. (All negligible for carbs.)

Totals: Day 3

Calories – 1974 kCal

Carbs – 44.33 grams

Protein – 108.9 grams

Day 4: Ketogenic meal suggestions

Breakfast: Day 4

Food	Protein (grams)	Carbohydrate (grams)	Calories (kCal)
Alpro strawberry and rhubarb yoghurt (150 grams)	5.4	14.1	111
Mix in 150 grams sunflower seeds	31.5	16.5	876
1 slice of PK bread (see page 21) (Approx. amounts)	5.0	0.5	125
Total	41.9	31.1	1112

Lunch: Day 4

Food	Protein (grams)	Carbohydrate (grams)	Calories(kCal)
Tinned ham (125 gram tin)	13.75	1.38	140
2 avocados (say 200 grams)	4.0	4.0	320
Frozen berries from freezer – 50 grams of raspberries	0.6	2.5	26
Total	18.35	7.88	486

Mid-afternoon snack: Day 4 (but try to avoid snacking)

Food	Protein (grams)	Carbohydrate (grams)	Calories (kCal)
Serious Pig salami (25 grams) (see page 18)	8.0	0.0	106
Total	8.0	0.0	106

Supper: Day 4

Food	Protein (grams)	Carbohydrate (grams)	Calories (kCal)
Tinned sardines in tomato juice (125 gram tin)	21.25	1.9	178
50 grams each of tomato,	0.45	1.35	9
cucumber,	0.7	0.8	8
lettuce	0.35	1.65	8
Dollop salad cream (say, 20 grams) (see page 59)	0.3	4.8	67
Total	23.05	10.5	270

Drinks: Day 4

Sparkling water as necessary; maximum of three cups of tea / coffee. (All negligible for carbs.)

Totals: Day 4

Calories – 1977 kCal

Carbs – 49.48 grams

Protein – 91.3 grams

Day 5: Ketogenic meal suggestions

Breakfast: Day 5

Food	Protein (grams)	Carbohydrate (grams)	Calories (kCal)
Coyo, pineapple, peach and passionfruit yoghurt (125 gram pot)	4.5	12.9	97
Mix in 100 grams sesame seeds	18.0	11.0	573
1 slice of PK bread (see page 21) (Approx. amounts)	5.0	0.5	125
With some cashew butter spread on this slice (say, 10 grams)	2.1	1.9	63
Total	29.6	26.3	858

Lunch: Day 5

Food	Protein (grams)	Carbohydrate (grams)	Calories (kCal)
Tinned red salmon (150 grams)	30.6	Trace	227
50 grams each of tomato,	0.45	1.35	9
cucumber,	0.7	0.8	8
lettuce	0.35	1.65	8
Dollop mayonnaise (20 grams) (see page 59)	0.2	Trace	136
Hazelnuts (10 grams)	1.5	0.7	63
Total	33.8	4.5	451

Mid-afternoon snack: Day 5 (but try to avoid snacking)

Food	Protein (grams)	Carbohydrate (grams)	Calories (kCal)
90% Lindt dark chocolate (50 grams)	5.0	8.25	297
Total	5.0	8.25	297

Supper: Day 5

Food	Protein (grams)	Carbohydrate (grams)	Calories (kCal)
Milano salami (75 grams)	18.6	0.38	260
Sauerkraut (200 grams)	1.4	2.8	38
Total	20.0	3.18	298

Drinks: Day 5

Sparkling water as necessary; maximum of three cups of tea / coffee. (All negligible for carbs.)

Totals: Day 5

> Calories – 1904 kCal
>
> Carbs – 42.23 grams
>
> Protein – 88.4 grams

Day 6: Ketogenic meal suggestions

Breakfast: Day 6

Food	Protein (grams)	Carbohydrate (grams)	Calories (kCal)
Alpro vanilla yoghurt (150 grams)	5.55	14.25	112
Mix in 100 grams flax seed	18.0	2.0	534
1 slice of PK bread (see page 21) (Approx. amounts)	5.0	0.5	125
With some coconut butter spread on this slice (say, 10 grams)	0.7	0.7	67
Total	29.25	17.45	838

Lunch: Day 6

Food	Protein (grams)	Carbohydrate (grams)	Calories (kCal)
Corned beef (125 gram tin)	31.0	1.38	282
50 grams each of tomato,	0.45	1.35	9
cucumber,	0.7	0.8	8
lettuce	0.35	1.65	8
Dollop mayonnaise (say, 10 grams) (see page 59)	0.1	Trace	68
Pine nuts (20 grams)	2.8	1.9	135
Total	35.4	7.08	510

Mid-afternoon snack: Day 6 (but try to avoid snacking)

Food	Protein (grams)	Carbohydrate (grams)	Calories (kCal)
Brazil nuts (40 grams)	5.6	1.6	262
Total	5.6	1.6	262

Supper: Day 6

Food	Protein (grams)	Carbohydrate (grams)	Calories (kCal)
Cornish pilchards in tomato sauce (120 gram tin)	17.4	2.88	190
One avocado (say, 100 grams)	2.0	2.0	160
Sauerkraut (200 grams)	1.4	2.8	38
Total	20.8	7.68	388

Drinks: Day 6

Sparkling water as necessary; maximum of three cups of tea / coffee. (All negligible for carbs.)

Totals: Day 6

Calories – 1998 kCal

Carbs – 33.81 grams

Protein – 91.05 grams

Day 7: Ketogenic meal suggestions

Breakfast: Day 7

Food	Protein (grams)	Carbohydrate (grams)	Calories (kCal)
Alpro soya yoghurt, plain (150 grams)	6.0	3.15	75
Mix with 100 grams chia seeds	17.0	8.0	486
1 slice of PK bread (see page 21) (Approx. amounts)	5.0	0.5	125
With some macadamia nut butter spread on this slice (say, 10 gram)	2.0	1.35	70
Pine nuts (20 grams)	2.8	1.9	135
Total	32.8	14.9	891

Lunch: Day 7

Food	Protein (grams)	Carbohydrate (grams)	Calories (kCal)
Chopped pork (200 gram tin)	33.8	1.2	414
50 grams each of tomato,	0.45	1.35	9
cucumber,	0.7	0.8	8
lettuce	0.35	1.65	8
Frozen berries from freezer – 50 grams of gooseberries	0.45	2.85	22
Total	35.75	7.85	461

Mid-afternoon snack: Day 7 (but try to avoid snacking)

Food	Protein (grams)	Carbohydrate (grams)	Calories (kCal)
Walnuts (50 grams)	7.5	3.5	327
Total	7.5	3.5	327

Supper: Day 7

Food	Protein (grams)	Carbohydrate (grams)	Calories (kCal)
Tinned tuna in spring water (120 grams)	32.4	Trace	135
50 grams each of tomato,	0.45	1.35	9
cucumber,	0.7	0.8	8
lettuce	0.35	1.65	8
Dollop mayonnaise (say, 10 grams) (see page 59)	0.1	Trace	68
Sauerkraut (200 grams)	1.4	2.8	38
Total	35.4	6.60	266

Drinks: Day 7

Sparkling water as necessary; maximum of three cups of tea / coffee. (All negligible for carbs.)

Totals: Day 7

Calories – 1945 kCal

Carbs – 32.85 grams

Protein – 111.45 grams

Appendix 6
Recommended products and suppliers

Amazon for:
Ketostix (www.amazon.co.uk/Ketostix-Reagent-Strips-Urinalysis-Ketone/dp/
B0000532GJ/ref=sr_1_1_a_it?ie=UTF8&qid=1469721894&sr=8-1&keywords=ketostix)

PK foods in Chapter 2
Bute Island (www.buteisland.com) for
Vegusto vegan cheese

Goodness Direct (www.goodnessdirect.co.uk) for
Sauerkraut (www.goodnessdirect.co.uk/cgi-local/frameset/script/search.
html?query=sauerkraut&snar)

Dr Myhill Co Ltd (www.sales@drmyhill.co.uk) for
Sunshine salt
Kefir culture – freeze-dried sachets

Natural Health Worldwide (www.naturalhealthworldwide.com) for tests and
consultations with health care professionals

Ocado for
foods listed in Chapter 2

Soil Association for
organic vegetable box schemes (www.soilassociation.org/organic-living/buy-
organic/find-an-organic-box-scheme/)

Tea Lyra (www.tealyra.co.uk) for
herbal teas

Appendix 7
The Dr Myhill Facebook group's version of PK bread

This slightly adapted version of the PK Bread recipe was developed by Queenie Eydís of Dr Myhill's Facebook Group; many members of that group have found that this recipe is easier to do and produces a loaf that rises particularly well.

- 250 g freshly ground organic linseed (as per Dr Myhill's instructions, see page 23-24)
- 270 ml freshly boiled water
- 1 tsp Sunshine Salt or Himalayan salt.
- 2 slightly heaped tablespoons psyllium husk powder (must be powder, not whole husks)

Heat the oven to at least 220°C
Grease a 0.454 kg (1 lb) loaf tin (as per Dr Myhill's instructions on page 24)
Place the freshly ground linseed and salt in a large bowl
Add the psyllium husk powder and mix well
Measure out the freshly boiled water and add to the linseed mix, quickly to activate the psyllium husk powder; the mixture will resemble play dough.
Mould the dough into a loaf shape with your hands and place in the prepared tin
Bake in the oven for 50 minutes to one hour
Turn out and cool; allow to cool before cutting

Notes:
Suma linseed is recommended
Don't try to grind whole psyllium husks into powder as this does not work as well as the pre-ground powder.

References

Chapter 1 – Why we should all be eating a PK diet

1. Dawkin R. *The Selfish Gene* 4th edition. Oxford University Press, Oxford, UK: 2016.

Chapter 3 – PK bread

1. Allaby RG, Peterson GW, Merriwether DA, Fu YB. Evidence of the domestication history of flax (*Linum usitatissimum L.*) from genetic diversity of the sad2 locus. *Theor Appl Genet* 2005; 112(1): 58-65. Epub 8 October 2005. (www.ncbi.nlm.nih. gov/pubmed/16215731)
2. Hirst KK. The eight founder crops and the origins of agriculture. *Thought Co* updated 13 November 2006 (www.thoughtco.com/founder-crops-origins-of-agriculture-171203 - accessed 20 April 2017)

Chapter 4 – PK dairy

1. Obituary: Dr Honor Anthony. Leeds University Secretariat 20 April 2011. (www. leeds.ac.uk/secretariat/obituaries/2011/anthony_honor.html – accessed 20 April 2017)
2. Lactose intolerance by ethnicity and region. ProCon.org. (http://milk.procon. org/view.resource.php?resourceID=000661 – accessed 20 April 2017)
3. Green J, Cairns BJ, Casabonne D, Wright FL, Reeves G, Beral V. Height and cancer incidence in the Million Women Study: prospective cohort, and meta-analysis of prospective studies of height and total cancer risk. *Lancet Oncology* 2011; 12(8): 785-794. doi: 10.1016/S1470-2045(11)70154-1
4. Gerstein HC. Cow's milk exposure and type 1 diabetes mellitus. A critical overview of the clinical literature. *Diabetes Care* 1994; 17(1): 13-19.
5. Virtanen SM, Rasanen L, Ylonen et al. Early introduction of dairy products associated with increased risk of IDDM in Finnish children. *Diabetes* 1993; 42(12):

1786-1790. doi.org/10.2337/diab.42.12.1786

6. Moss M, Freed D. The cow and the coronary: epidemiology, biochemistry and immunology. *International Journal of Cardiology* 2003; 87(2-3): 203-216. (www.ncbi. nlm.nih.gov/pubmed/12559541)

Chapter 5 – PK breakfasts

1. Ichinose-Kuwahara T, Inoue Y, Iseki Y, Hara S, Ogura, Kondo N. Sex differences in the effects of physical training on sweat gland responses during a graded exercise. *Experimental Physiology* 2010; 10: 1026-1032. doi: 10.1113/expphysiol.2010.053710

2. Alleyne R. Men perspire and women glow, science proves. *The Telegraph* 8 October 2010. (http://www.telegraph.co.uk/news/health/news/8048508/Men-perspire-and-women-glow-science-proves.html – accessed 20 April 2017)

3. Bredersen DE. Reversal of cognitive decline: a novel therapeutic approach. *Aging* 2014; 6(9): 707-717. (www.impactaging.com)

Chapter 7 – PK main courses – soups, stews and roasts

1. Fallon SA. Broth is beautiful. Weston A Price Foundation 1 January 2000. (www. westonaprice.org/health-topics/broth-is-beautiful/ –accessed 20 April 2017)

Chapter 8 – PK salads

1. Spence C. Eating with our ears: assessing the importance of the sounds of consumption on our perception and enjoyment of multisensory flavour experiences. *Flavour* 3 March 2015. doi: 10.1186/2044-7248-4-3

Chapter 9 – Lard, dripping and fat

1. Fernandez C. We're not telling porkies… happy pigs oink more! Animals' grunts and squeals show off their personalities and how content they are in their pens. *Daily Mail* 29 June 2016. (http://www.dailymail.co.uk/sciencetech/article-3665092/We-not-telling-porkies-happy-pigs-oink-Animals-grunts-squeals-help-personalities-content-pens.html – accessed 20 April 2017)

Chapter 10 – Sweeteners

1. Lally P, Jaarsveld CHM van, Potts HWW. How are habits formed: Modelling habit formation in the real world. *European Journal of Social Psychology* 2010; 40(6): 998–1009. doi:10.1002/ejsp.674

2. Rycerz K, Jaworska-Adamu JE. Effects of aspartame metabolites on astrocytes and neurons. *Folia Neuropathol* 2013; 51(1): 10-17. (www.ncbi.nlm.nih.gov/pubmed/23553132)

3. Soffritti M, Padovani M, Tibaldi E, Falcioni L, Manservisi F, Belpoggi F. The carcinogenic effects of aspartame: the urgent need for regulatory re-evaluation. *Am J Ind Med* 2014; 57(4): 383-397. doi: 10.1002/ajim.22296. Epub 2014 Jan 16. (www.ncbi.nlm.nih.gov/pubmed/24436139)

4. Milchovich S, Dunn-Long B. *Diabetes Mellitus: A Practical Handbook* 10th edition. Bull Publishing Company, 2011, page 79.

5. Ford-Martin P, Blumer I. *The Everything Diabetes Book* 1st edition. Everything Books, 2004, page 124.

Chapter 11 – Herbs and spices

1. Schwartz K, Chang HT, Nikolai M, et al. Treatment of glioma patients with ketogenic diets: report of two cases treated with an IRB-approved energy-restricted ketogenic diet protocol and review of the literature. *Cancer & Metabolism* 2015; 3: 3. doi: 10.1186/s40170-015-0129-1

2. Carbone I, Lazzarotto T, Ianni M, et al. Herpes virus in Alzheimer's disease: relation to progression of the disease. *Neurobiology of Aging* 2014; 35(1): 122-129. doi: 10.1016/j.neurobiolaging.2013.06.024

3. Libby P, Egan D, Skariatos S. Roles of infectious agents in atherosclerosis and restenosis: an assessment of the evidence needed for future research. *Circulation* 1997; 96: 4095-4103. doi: 10.1161/01.CIR.96.11.4095

4. American Cancer Society. Infections that can lead to cancer – get an overview of how infections with some viruses, bacteria, and other germs may increase a person's risk for certain types of cancer. ACS. (www.cancer.org/cancer/cancer-causes/infectious-agents/infections-that-can-lead-to-cancer.html – accessed 20 April 2017)

5. Buettner D. The island where people forget to die. *The New York Times Magazine*.

24 October 2012. (www.nytimes.com/2012/10/28/magazine/the-island-where-people-forget-to-die.html?_r=0 – accessed 20 April 2017)

6. Shehzad A, Rehman G, Lee YS. Curcumin in inflammatory diseases. *Biofactors* 2013; 39(1): 69-77. doi: 10.1002/biof.1066

7. Kaefer CM, Milner JA. The Role of Herbs and Spices in Cancer Prevention. *J Nutr Biochem* 2008; 19(6): 347–361. doi: 10.1016/j.jnutbio.2007.11.003

8. Kaefer CM, Milner JA. Herbs and Spices in Cancer Prevention and Treatment. In: Benzie IFF, Wachtel-Gaylor S. *Herbal Medicine: Biomolecular and Clinical Aspects* 2nd edition. CRC Press/Taylor & Francis: 2011. (www.ncbi.nlm.nih.gov/books/NBK92774/ – accessed 20 April 2017)

Chapter 12 – Fermented foods

1. Chilton SN et al (2015) Inclusion of Fermented Foods in Food Guides around the World. *Nutrients* 2015; 7(1): 390–404. (www.ncbi.nlm.nih.gov/pmc/articles/PMC4303846/ – accessed 20 April 2017)

2. Grass G, Rensing C, Solioz M. Metallic copper as an antimicrobial surface. *Applied Environmental Microbiology* 2011; 77(5): 1541–1547. (www.ncbi.nlm.nih.gov/pmc/articles/PMC3067274/ – accessed 20 April 2017)

3. The Copper Development Association. Copper kills antibiotic-resistant "nightmare bacteria" – antimicrobial copper products in hospitals should be considered as a response to CDC's latest warning on lethal bacteria. *PR Newswire* 12 March 2013. (www.prnewswire.com/news-releases/copper-kills-antibiotic-resistant-nightmare-bacteria-197333411.html – accessed 20 April 2017)

4. WHO. World Health Statistics 2016: Monitoring health for the SDGs Annex B: tables of health statistics by country, WHO region and globally. World Health Organization, 2016. (www.who.int/gho/publications/world_health_statistics/2016/Annex_B/en/ – accessed 20 April 2017)

Chapter 13 – Sunshine minerals

1. Eisenberg MJ. Magnesium deficiency and sudden death. *American Heart Journal* 1992; 124(2): 544-549.

2. Nielsen FH, Lukaski HC. Update on the relationship between magnesium and exercise. *Magnes Research* 2006; 19(3): 180-189.

3. Mayer A-M. Historical changes in the mineral content of fruits and vegetables. *British Food Journal* 1997; 99(6): 207-211. doi: 10.1108/00070709710181540

4. McCance RA, Widdowson EM. *The Composition of Foods* Third edition. Medical Research Council Special Report series No. 213, HMSO, London, 1960.

5. Holland B, Welch AA, Unwin ID, Buss DH, Paul AA, Southgate DAT. *McCance and Widdowson's Composition of Foods* Fifth edition. Royal Society of Chemistry and the Ministry of Agriculture, Fisheries and Food, HMSO, London, 1991.

6. Lindlahr. *Nature Cure; Philosophy and Practice Based on the Unity of Disease and Cure..* 1914

7. Hamaker. *The Survival of Civilization*. 1982.

8. USDA. *USDA Agriculture Handbook No. 8: Composition of Foods... Raw, processed, prepared*. 1963

9. Watt and Merrill *Home Economics Research Report No. 54: Nutrient Content of the U.S. Food Supply, 1909-97*. 1997.

Chapter 14 – PK water

1. Buck B. Don't drink the (warm) water left in a plastic bottle, UF/IFAS study says. *IFAS News* 22 September 2014. http://news.ifas.ufl.edu/2014/09/dont-drink-the-warm-water-ufifas-study-says/ (Accessed 25 April 2017)

2. Fan Y-Y, Zheng J-L, Ren J-H, Luo J, Ma LQ. Effects of storage temperature and duration on release of antimony and bisphenol A from polythene terephthalate drinking bottles of China. *Environmental Pollution* 2014; 192: 113-120. doi.org/10.1016/j.envpol.2014.05.012

Appendix 3 – Carb values

1. United States Department of Agriculture (USDA) – Agricultural Research Service (ARS). USDA National Nutrient Database for Standard Reference: Release 28. USDA; 18 August 2016. (https://www.ars.usda.gov/northeast-area/beltsville-md/beltsville-human-nutrition-research-center/nutrient-data-laboratory/docs/usda-national-nutrient-database-for-standard-reference/ – accessed 20 April 2017)

Appendix 4 – Nutritional supplements for the PK diet

1. Marler JB, Wallin JR. Nutrition Security Institute White Paper: Human Health, the Nutritional Quality of Harvested Food and Sustainable Farming Systems. Nutrition Security Institute, 2006. (www.nutritionsecurity.org/PDF/NSI_White%20Paper_Web.pdf – accessed 20 April 2017)

Index

Postscript

Western Medicine has lost its way. Doctors no longer look for the underlying causes of disease, a process which used to be called diagnosis, but rather seek a 'quick fix' response that will see the patient out of their surgery door in under 10 minutes. This quick fix response usually comprises the prescribing of symptom-suppressing medications. Doctors have become the puppets of Big Pharma, dishing out drugs and working to a 'checklist' culture which is directed at the symptom, rather than the patient. Patients are seen as a collection of walking symptoms, rather than as people, each with a highly individual set of circumstances. Worse than this, not only do these prescription drugs do nothing to address the root causes of illness, but often they accelerate the underlying pathology and so drug prescribing snowballs. This leads to a vicious spiral of increasing drug costs, coupled with worsening pathologies for individual patients, whilst at the same time there is an increasing number of new, and chronic, patients, because their illnesses are never properly addressed at the root cause. It is no wonder that the National Health Service is being overwhelmed. The result is that millions suffer a painful, premature, and often lingering, death from diseases which are completely avoidable and reversible.

The time has come for patients to be empowered, by taking back control of their own health. To achieve this empowerment, patients need:

1. The knowledge to work out why they have symptoms and disease.
2. Direct access to all relevant medical tests.
3. Direct access to knowledgeable health practitioners who can further advise and guide patients, together with direct access to safe and effective remedies.

None of this is beyond patients who are always highly motivated to be well again, and who always know their bodies better than anyone else. It is time to break down the artificial barriers that have been placed between patients and direct access to the medical knowledge, tests and experts that they so deserve.

This three-stage process of patient emancipation is addressed in the following ways.

1. The knowledge can be found in these five books

a) *Sustainable Medicine* - This is the starting point for treating all symptoms and diseases. It explains why we have symptoms, such as fatigue and pain, and explains how we can work out the mechanisms of such symptoms and which are the appropriate medical tests for diagnosing these mechanisms. Most importantly, *Sustainable Medicine* identifies the 'tools of the trade' to affect a cure. These tools include diet, nutritional supplements and natural remedies.

b) *Prevent & Cure Diabetes – delicious diets not dangerous drugs*. All medical therapies should start with diet. Modern Western diets are driving our modern epidemics of diabetes, heart disease, cancer and dementia; this process is called metabolic syndrome. *Prevent & Cure Diabetes* explains in detail why and how we have arrived at a situation where the *real* weapons of mass destruction can be found in our kitchens. Importantly, it describes the vital steps every one of us can make to reverse this situation so that life can be lived to its full potential.

c) *Diagnosis & Treatment of Chronic Fatigue Syndrome and Myalgic Encephalitis – it's mitochondria not hypochondria*. This book further explores the commonest symptom which people complain of, namely fatigue, together with its pathological end result when this symptom is ignored. This is Dr Myhill's life work, having spent over 35 years in clinical practice, many months of academic research and the co-authoring of three scientific papers, all directed at solving this jigsaw puzzle of an illness. This book has application not just for the severely fatigued patient but also for the athlete looking for peak performance.

d) *The PK Cookbook*. This gives us the *how* of the 'PK' diet that the other books conclude is essential. It is the starting point for preventing and treating modern Western diseases, including diabetes, arterial disease, dementia and cancer. Dietary changes are always the most difficult, but also the most important, intervention. This book is based on Dr Myhill's first-hand experience and research into developing a PK diet that is sustainable long term. Perhaps the most important feature of this diet is the PK bread – this has helped more people stick to this diet than all else! Secondly, Dr Myhill introduces PK salt (named 'sunshine salt' because it is rich in vitamin D). This salt is comprised of all essential minerals (plus vitamins D and B12) in physiological amounts within a sea salt. This more than compensates for the mineral deficiencies that are ubiquitously present in all foods from Western agricultural systems. It is an essential and delicious addition to all modern Western diets.

e) *The Natural Treatment of Infection – Life is an Arms Race*. This tells us why modern life is an Arms Race and which infections are driving Western diseases. It also details why we are losing this Arms Race and the clinical signs and symptoms that demonstrate this. Then comes the good news! There are chapters detailing the general approach to fighting infections and then also specific measures for specific infections, including EBV (glandular fever, 'mono'), Lyme disease, bartonella and others. How to diagnose these infections is also covered and there are special sections on how to treat acute infections and also how to protect your microbiome. The vast majority of the approaches in this book are natural, including many herbal preparations, and can be done by readers completely on their own, with no need to involve doctors. Prescription medications are reserved only for intransigent cases. Finally, you will learn about the unique 'groundhog' protocol for promoting and maintaining good health.

2. Access to medical tests

Many medical tests can be accessed directly through

https://www.bloodtestsdirect.co.uk/ where blood tests can be accessed directly without a doctor's request. Many can be done on fingerdrop samples of blood.

http://www.arminlabs.com/en blood tests can be accessed directly without the need for a referral form a doctor or health practitioner.

http://www.biolab.co.uk/ (needs referral from a health practitioner — see 'NHW' below)

https://www.gdx.net/uk/ (Genova labs for stool, urine and saliva testing – needs referral from a health practitioner - see 'NHW' below). Tests include blood, urine, stool and saliva samples. Many blood tests can be carried out at home on a fingerdrop sample of blood, without the need for a nurse or doctor to be involved at all.

3. Direct access to knowledgeable practitioners who can further advise and guide patients

Natural Health Worldwide (NHW) is a website where any knowledgeable practitioner (medical doctor, health professional or experienced patient) can offer their opinion to any patient. This opinion may be free, or for a fee, by telephone, email, Skype or

Facetime. The practitioner needs no premises or support staff since bookings and payments are made online. Patients give feedback to that practitioner's 'Reputation page' and star ratings evolve. See www.naturalhealthworldwide.com